To Wendy McAuslan

HELLO TO YOU

A wise person, compared to me, said that if people are going to want to read this book then you need to do an introduction so that anyone new to you and your world will quickly know whether they want to read on; a way of checking if the blurb on the back cover lives up to its promise.

This is a musing, a meandering through real life. It is not about drama, although there is drama. It is not about devastation, although there is devastation. This is a book about living, about understanding, about learning, about growing, about love and also grief, about summers walking the dog by the sea and winters when we are too tired to think. It is about answering the alarm when the world is so surreal and dark that school and work seem like an absurdity and because it is me, it is about the world of mental illness and compulsory treatment and trying to live a normal life when everyone says there is no such thing as normal.

It is almost not a book; I have learnt very late in life that there is something wrong with the compartments in which I place my identity; there is my mental illness, my compulsory treatment, my new family, my work, the family I grew up with and still love very much, there is death, love, sex, there is boredom and a drive to succeed and change the world even though I no longer know how to change the world or why. There is a cliché associated with each one and a stereoptype which I have taken to heart. My book is divided into its different subjects like a calendar or an essay. You can read all about my feelings for Wendy, you can find out about life with grief and work in lockdown, mental illness and mental health, my dad and Wendy's dad and finally, all the bits we all carry on doing whatever the dramas are that are going on around us. I don't know any other way of placing these parts of my life together because, although they are all part of me they are separate, maybe as I meander through, the sections will meld together, different bits speak to each other.

The book is not all sad. In fact there are some funny bits. It is about my dad, and Wendy's dad's illness and their deaths but also it is about family. It does not try to make you think in a certain way about living or dying, family or work and how we approach it. I tell my tale as it happened to me and those I love.

We will all die, and most of us will fall in love and feel the joy and fear of new relationships. Most of us will wake up after that first wonderful rush of love and find the world different. Many of us nowadays find ourselves in relationships where the children in the family are not our children and have to learn how to navigate that rich, complex and terrifying world.

*

Why do I feel I have the right to write about such things? I am not sure I do. However, I know that, all appearances to the contrary, in the real world, where I am known for my silence, that I have a lot to say and it is as simple as that: I want to tell you bits of this story.

I think I may bring something special because what we all go through when we die or witness loved ones die or when we fall in love, is special. What you go through; what your friends go through; that is special too. I love to hear of people's different worlds, whether that is in books, on film, in the pub or on a walk and I hope you will like and be interested in the glimpses I give you into my world.

I bring a very, very, niche perspective of the anxieties that occur when someone who has a mental illness tries to develop and sustain a life-long, loving relationship. But maybe there are connections to others who are also taking that step into the bonds of family and love. I may give an even more niche perspective to those people who stand on the edge of tragedy and who desperately want to help those they love, but doubt they have the skills to do so; maybe here there are some tips for people like me who are trying to help the people they love with something so difficult.

You can read about the years before I moved down to Argyll, in *START*, my memoir about my years of breakdowns, the harshness of my marriage and the beauty of falling in love with Wendy. This new book is a continuation of those years, it tells tales of some of the things that have happened since *START*.

If any of this appeals to you, do read on. I will be glad of your company.

January

2020—JANUARY—WENDY—ONE DAY I WILL NOT NEED TO WRITE THESE THINGS DOWN

Palette of grey and white. A walk from the shore.

It slips away into the mist, a long silent glide and then away. I am not sure what it was: a gull of some sort. Hand in hand we walk on the mud and sand, shrouded in the grey white of the fog. Gulls, oystercatchers, crows and curlews stand silently at the water's rim. As we approach, they lift off, disappear into the whiteness to settle further along the firth's edge, or behind us, at the patch of water and sand we have just left.

Here the world is muffled, quiet, ethereal. The land merges into the sea, merges into the sky. Motion is a hushed surprise. The far off, soft sound of children laughing somewhere behind the whiteness on the path, near where the horses graze, reinforces just how closed in this world of fog is, on the shore at Ardmore.

I had wanted to wander up above Cardross; to walk in the hills where the sky was bright and the grass spiky with the glint of frost but Wendy said, "Let's go down into the fog and see what it is like."

It is a world of silver, of shaded contrasts, where the sun shining through the sea's clouds makes the world opaque but so bright. The ripples in the sand cast grey shadows that ease into the water between them. The tiny, almost imperceptible, lip and lap of the sea eases into the beach. We have wandered hundreds of metres from the shore, through pools of water that are so shallow they are not quite pools, over ridges of sand that are so small they are not quite ridges. The only breach of the smoothness is the sudden appearance of old cockle shells, the ubiquitous casts of the worms in the sand.

Wendy walks out into the sea in her wellies with Dash the dog beside her on his lead. The water splashes under them, makes its own concentric pattern. The birds lift off around them; vanish. The sea is so shallow that it seems as though we are walking constantly to a nowhere, with no beginning and no ending to the shore, the sand, the pools of the world we have found ourselves in.

Back at the dry shore, the wonder changes when we find an old bare sculpture of driftwood standing high from a tree stump. Jewelled strands of seaglass hang from blue polypropylene ropes, old metal buckets, abandoned blue hard hats, heaps of shells, seaweed and old broken dolls, so many different coloured ropes from which the flotsam dangles. Mounds of crockery line the base and all around us is the stillness of the mist; the coldness of the ice of the water frozen along the shore.

We walk hand in hand again, along the shore, lost in the awe of something very special that we hadn't expected, back to cuddles at home; telly, coffee and slow conversation, punctuated with laughter at the wonder of where we have just been.

2021—JANUARY—MY JOURNAL

Coming back to work after around three months off is a strange feeling. I still don't really know what it is that made me shudder to a halt. It may have been the horrible people on the internet who have been so incredibly harsh to me and Wendy over the years, or the long year of working from home during Covid, and it must have been my dad's death. You do not take sick leave on the very anniversary of his funeral, a year ago, without it being connected in some way, do you? It has made me reflect on these last few years with Wendy: my new family, my new job, the helter-skelter of all that has been going on since I drove up to her door with all my possessions packed into my car.

When I arrived at Wendy's for our new life together, I thought that I had reached the end of a fairy tale and that it would continue in the way fairy tales are meant to; that life would start bright, fresh, with laughing lovable children, kisses, cuddles and, of course, the birds singing and the butterflies flapping idly in the never-ending summer sunshine.

I wrote all about my loneliness and sadness in my book, *START*. I went into detail about my diagnosis of schizophrenia and my continuing compulsory treatment, the break-up of my marriage, my estrangement from my son; all these things.

But although that story finished with the excitement I felt when, as part of my new job, I was due to speak to the United Nations Committee against Torture about the detention of people like me, it also finished with what I thought was realism. I knew my compulsory treatment would likely continue. I knew life was not always rosy, even with my new family, and said so. I even went down that traditional route of making the point that life is never smooth and that people like me are not dignified with the labels of tragedy, victimhood or heroism.

Wendy and I had talked about our future and realised that we could not alternate weekends between Nairn and Cardross when my drive to her took over four hours and her bus journey well over six hours. And anyway, we wanted more than weekends together.

This was to be our new start; our beginning. I really did think the deer would pause as I drove past them and look at my smiling face with a knowing look, a hint of a blessing. I thought that now everything would be wonderful. I knew it wouldn't be, but I thought it would be, despite that. After all, I was in love with someone who loved me. I adored her young children who also seemed to like me, and hadn't I given up my job, my house, the rich network of friends I had in the Highlands to start my new life? Of course we deserved something wonderful!

And it has been wonderful.

Except, Wendy's dad was dying of cancer. My dad had Parkinson's disease. My niece attempted suicide and, like me, was sectioned. My sister was recovering from the aftermath of her house burning down and was trying to start her own new life with her family in Scotland, as a midwife. Wendy had to have an operation for endometriosis and had to deal with some particularly unpleasant people and politics at work. James, her son, was admitted to the Intensive Care Unit of the Sick Kids in Glasgow, with Ludwig's Angina, and I still had my whatever it is; my schizophrenia, my depression, my anxiety and the enormous quantity of alcohol I drank every night. The children – they had to watch their beloved Papa, as they called their grandad (Sandy), die, and had to adjust to my presence, which happened with varying levels of success.

So now, over six years later, with both our dads now dead, it seems like we have been in some desperate conflict; that as a family we have washed up on the shore; panting, shattered, saying to each other, "How on earth did we survive that?"

Because we do seem to have, except there are no happy endings so far. I still think we need a happy ending and a chance to just stop and say, "Well, that was a bit shit! Let's do something different and a great deal more fun."

And I don't even swear! Wendy will be shocked when she reads this. Of course, we won't do something so much more fun because fairy tales, when we leave Disney behind, are often pretty grim and about lives which are also so often grim and dark.

Despite the blessing our life can be, I still have schizophrenia; we have mothers who are growing older, friends and relations with their own tragedies. That is how it is for most people: lightness obscured by the difficulty of living.

Despite that, when we pause in the evening, we know that, compared to many people, including many people we know, we are indeed blessed; that to some people our life is a living fairy tale of the Disney sort, especially if you look at all my Instagram posts of flowers and hills, Dash the dog and walks by the sea.

I have tried to write about everything as it happened during the last few years and in recent months, I have gathered my words into a great puddle of stories and diary entries, but sadly for me, there are so many threads and different themes that I need to drain that puddle to give some clarity. I need to distil the messiness of our lives into just a few points so that the puddle runs clear, flows musically down the hill.

If you have ever been on a writing course you will have heard all these entreaties to 'Show not Tell'. But to some extent I do want to tell. I want you to see a tiny delicate family growing and grieving. I want to show you glimpses of life; like walking in the snow and laughing, when the next day we will hear the results of Sandy's latest tests. I want you to see me waiting for the train, almost oblivious to the everyday tragedy we are experiencing. Above all, I want you to see us getting the children ready for school: Wendy dressing them, me making their breakfast and packing their bags and making their lunch when their Papa has only weeks left to live, because that is the reality of tragedy. We still make lunch, go to work, fill the car with petrol, do the shopping. Or at least, that is reality for some people. That was our reality.

These three months off have been a revelation. I have never ever taken time off in such a major way before, unless it has been done against my will. A part of me thinks that for the first time I have been able to take responsibility for my mental health.

I find that slightly frightening; the thought of actually engaging with those who help me, the thought of maybe one day acknowledging properly this schizophrenia thing. I look at Twitter and Facebook and Instagram a lot and find myself alien, even from the people who experience psychosis. They seem so aware, so in touch with the foibles of life and perception, so busy working out how to improve their lives and talk with their therapists. Just the fact that they refer to doctors as therapists bamboozles me. I report to my nurse and am summoned to see my doctor, and occasionally I break some of my silence and confide bits of my existence, but to participate and engage? Maybe it is a British and an American thing? Maybe their experience is very different to mine?

January has been a month of all sorts of things. My article on those months of sick leave appeared in *Mental Health Today* and I even got paid for it. It was so easy and fun to write and makes me wish I could make a career from writing, but even I know that is naïve. You will see the article later on in this chapter and maybe it will make you think a little.

Selected January highlights… I have started to dream about my dad. I hardly think about him and have rarely felt much emotion at all about his death. We talk about him a bit, usually to wonder what he and Sandy would have said if they had witnessed Covid or met each other, or to remember times when we visited him and Mum.

Nowadays, I often close my eyes late at night, befuddled a bit with tiredness and alcohol, and there he is, vivid and real again in my dreams. Often those dreams are nightmares and I wake sweaty and panicky. And yet, it is such a relief to see my dad when I sleep and to know that even if daytime me cannot grieve, that nighttime me is allowing, at last, that grief to bubble up and sweep away those feelings, to resolve the long months where I do not know what it is I think about him no longer being here; that sudden jolt when I phone my mum and am about to ask if Dad wants to speak and remember he will never do so again.

We got rabbits for Charlotte. That was exciting! Shortly after school started again, I converted Charlotte's upscaled toy cupboard into a rabbit hutch. Using the jig saw to cut away the doors was awful. I had assumed I would create straight lines, with the blades rushing through the thin wood, but instead they rattled and shuddered, with dust and splinters all over the place and very wobbly lines. The chicken wire was more fragile than I thought but good at jagging me, and the wood so hard that

I needed to drill holes to hammer the nails in and yes, of course, I did also hammer my fingers.

That Sunday we went down the village to Charlie's mum's house. Working out how to pass across cash and get rabbits, while socially distanced, seeing Charlotte and James rushing down the road with their dad to get to us in time to pick them up. The excitement at home of toffee-and-cream-coloured Pumpkin and black-furred Bonbon. Only Bonbon could get up the ramp to the second floor of their cage so I needed to fix some steps to it to make it accessible to Pumpkin too.

What else has January brought us? Walks in the cold, in the ice, in the mist, in the rain and the gales; they are such a wonderful break from lockdown.

Of course, the biggest bit was going back to home schooling again, now we are in the second lockdown again. It was so different to the last year's lockdown. Now the children sign in to Seesaw at nine, work through the lesson plan, attend Google Meets, work some more. In the spring we had vague instructions to count leaves and bumble bees; now we are doing times tables and division, literacy and PE and the children do not enjoy it! It is a rare day we get them to register before ten. A rare day that there is not some sort of meltdown at a lesson and a rare day that we do not have to tell them how rude it is to turn off Google Meets before the teacher has said goodbye. And combining home working with this? Almost impossible.

I would like to claim credit but cannot. Fond dreams of not being sexist quickly fell by the wayside. James point-blank refused to work with me, would hide under his blanket and wail. Charlotte did co-operate which was good. Wendy had set up all the apps and things and so she was the person every morning who set out the lesson plan, worked out who would do what; made sure we were all in the house for the meet up. Dealt with the morning, "I hate my school, I hate my teacher!" tantrums. I helped.

I helped.

What a pathetic word! I made things easier. As usual, I did the cooking, shopping, cleaning and things but I never ran a complete day's class without Wendy having to play a part and I frequently absented myself to take Zoom and Teams calls, to write my speeches and reports. I didn't have such a frantic juggling of work and school and dogs and children; a fair amount of it but nothing approaching what Wendy went through. Sometimes she would be so tired at the end of the day.

I got sectioned again, as is usual at this time of year. The casualness of it does shock me. I knew my psychiatrist would need to be thinking about renewing my CTO sometime around now, but sitting, waiting for my appointment, with my face mask on, my hands cleaned from the container by reception, only for him to say we would be meeting in the conference room and that my MHO would be there and a student. What is that? Thirty seconds notice that they would be deciding whether to renew it; no preparation, no nothing! Still that is the way it is, I can't be bothered to get indignant.

Wendy is glad that I am thinking about my dad more, glad that I took time off work. She was saying, not long ago, that she has to reach so far to get through to me. That despite the confessional nature of Twitter and Instagram, she rarely knows what I am really thinking or feeling and needs to search for the real me amongst my silence, my aversion from feelings and reality and expression.

I am incredibly lucky that she finds that relatively easy to do and knows from experience that it is maybe not just some sign of toxic masculinity that makes it so hard for me to speak.

So, now I am back at work, perched at the top of the house, doing my Teams calls, my Zoom calls. It is like I was never away and I am not sure how I feel about that. I resolved nothing about my dad while I was off, did not learn how to be spontaneous or creative with the children. I still find it hard to access the laughter and that joy I once had at life.

I still drink myself to sleep. I miss those afternoons when Wendy and I would sleep together, with no other thought than the pleasure of each other's company and the prospect of hours more curled up with laughter simmering.

2021—JANUARY—ALAN IDRIS MORGAN— RECOLLECTIONS

It is hard now that I come to talk of my dad. I don't want to claim some sort of repressed grief for him that I only find when I allow myself the luxury of sleep, but somehow that is how it feels. When I close my eyes nowadays, I am always half-expecting to find my dad there. Usually it is some innocuous dream, one of those where we are sailing over the Atlantic or something, one of the ones which Wendy says is one of 'those' dreams. Where I am journeying on a long, maybe lonely, maybe dangerous voyage; leaving my dad behind on land but still doing his bidding, taking one of his boats somewhere, either to sell it or take it to a boat show, something like that.

In other dreams, he walks ahead of us in a foreign Mediterranean city, so fast we cannot keep up, and me and my brother smile knowingly at each other, a typical *look at Dad!* look, but he turns into an alley. We see people following him, intent on harming him, and though we run as fast as we can, we cannot stop him being beaten up though we do restrain his attackers for future arrest.

I am pretty blind to symbolism or meaning but even I can imagine there is something in there about death and our journey through life and my relationship with my dad.

It took me a long time to realise I loved my dad. It will probably take even longer to know just how much now that he is dead. In my early years, my main memory is of him dressed in his RAF uniform at the breakfast table before setting off to Fighter Command or whatever it was he went to when we lived in Buckinghamshire. I was in awe of him and tried my very best to eat like he did, and definitely thought he came out best when the children on the estate we lived on compared the jobs their dads did. I remember him whistling in the car with my mum when we drove for what seemed like hours on the way to visit our grandparents, with their sweets, sweet-smelling house and sweet tea. I remember him chasing a car that splashed through a puddle and covered my mum in mud; chasing it, catching it and getting the money to dry clean her clothes. I remember the walks with the dog on the hill at Downley, in the setting sun of summer evenings. I remember him trying to teach us this special way of getting over gates where you grip it in such a way that your body seems to fly over it, and I remember how proud we were of his sailing and how he was in the newspapers, but that we did not see him much because he was either flying or at sea.

Then there is a sort of gap that spans many decades. It started when we were sent away to school when we were nine and ended, how long ago? Maybe fifteen years ago, maybe longer.

It is the gap where many of my memories have clouded themselves and where, from a distance, I piled up a huge pyramid of resentment that weighed me down and my family down and which, because it was so huge, became unmanageable and distorted my vision. For many, many years of my adulthood, when I should have known better, I used family get-togethers to get drunk with my brother and sister and say how awful Dad had been to us.

But there were wonderful times in those years; it is hard how the highlights dilute themselves. When we first started sailing it was a revelation, a terrifying revelation. We had always been to sea with Dad. Apparently, when I was six months old I fell out of my carry cot in the bows of some boat in a storm and landed in a coil of anchor rope and carried on sleeping, oblivious to the panic of the adults who couldn't find me! I remember, and strangely, I remember it in black and white, some sailing trip with us in a very muddy anchorage somewhere on the east coast. The clouds were grey and the yacht was dark and cold and my dad and someone else were drinking whisky. Whoever the someone else was, he was very funny and tried to see if I could sing, "I was born under a Wandering Star" in a lower voice than him.

But back to the terrifying revelation: sailing and finding out that boats tip up in the wind and that if you don't hold onto the stanchions, you will slip all the way across the cockpit into the sea. And however much the adults tell you the keel of a yacht stops it from being able to capsize, when you are out of sight of land on a sunny day and there is spray in the air you, or rather, I, can be convinced the boat will turn right over and will be holding on for dear life!

But those days of sunshine, with the wind in our faces and the brilliance of the sea, the wake behind us, Richard telling long complicated stories to Juliet; bread, cheese, fruit, wine and pâté in the cockpit and a berth to lie in down below when the sun makes us too hot and tired; where you can listen to the sound of the rigging, feel the sway and tip of the boat, smell some sort of mixture of sour milk and diesel from the bilges, and feel comfortable and safe.

We had so many holidays and weekends like that. They weren't all good. Sometimes there was a lot of noise and a lot of shouting. When we were older and played a bigger part in the actual sailing, I remember the kerfuffle if we led the sheets the wrong way along the decking, or if a spinnaker wrapped itself around the mast. Then, after the barrage of wind in the sails, the thundering of my dad, we would be silent and resentful but equally, I remember anchorages and meals in restaurants and the slight movement of the boat, the occasional click of the halyards. The fresh feel of the sea when we jumped into it and the rush of bubbles all around our bodies, trying to swim under the hull and up the other side; trying to remember sea shanties.

I remember the Thatched Cottage and Mrs Twiggy, the gardener, parties where my dad was loud and very, very happy. Visits from the Geoghegans at Christmas which were close to bliss, walks on the beach and some sort of weird flamethrower that we found in the shed and which, to our amazement, worked. Dad digging up the garden with a rotavator, the lovely wooden doors to the bedrooms, with wonderful catches. Watching the Lightnings flying offshore and thinking our dad was probably in one of them.

And after my son was born, how Dad prepared and prepared for each visit. How there were times my son went down there on his own, in the days when minors could fly alone on aeroplanes, and how Dad would have made a huge programme of visits to entertain him, or when we were all there, and my son walked along the row of peas, taking bites out of each pod, and how Charlie the dog would sit beside him for hours when he was asleep in his cot. There were some truly wonderful times. I find I am cross with myself because I only have a sketchy memory of them.

When I became more friendly with Mum and Dad, I would often fly down south to walk by the Seven Sisters with my mum and over towards Alfriston with her on sunny days.

As usual, the conversation would often be about my dad; his future, his retirement, his mood, his health. He was good at being a focal point. In some ways he was very good when he retired. He took it seriously and didn't do very much at all: reading a lot, doing his woodwork, sitting in the garden in the sun with a beer. Initially, he was very involved with the church, especially with its finances, but as time went by, he relaxed into something smooth.

His back pained him. He got prostate cancer which he recovered from. Sometimes we wondered if he was depressed because he did so little. His movements became more erratic until my brother's wife, Kathryn, who was a GP, suggested he get assessed for Parkinson's.

And that was the beginning of a slow loss. The visits north ebbed away slowly. There was one when he met my son for the last time. There was another where we toured Argyll rather than Highland, in which I remember vividly all of us pretending to be different types of bird while driving towards Bute and giggling uncontrollably. But his movement and control of his body became too difficult, and there came a time when he took to his mobility scooter and Wendy and I would fly down early in the morning for a few days every few months to see him and my mum.

For me they were good years.

For me, the smoothing out of my dad happened as he became more frail; that gentling and that smile and that affection was just what I needed. For my mum, maybe less so. I think she missed the vigour and the energy he once took to life; that seizing of each moment of the day, that capacity to charm and argue and do a myriad of different things.

I reflect on this more and more now that he is dead. I miss him. I don't really want to talk to him just now, but to sit in the garden under the sunshade with our lunch and our books while the pigeons call and the seagulls stalk around on top of the roof. That would be wonderful.

2021—JANUARY—ME AND MY MENTAL HEALTH—I TOOK THREE MONTHS OFF SICK BECAUSE OF MY MENTAL ILL HEALTH AND HAD THE MOST FUN IN AGES

Three and a half months ago, I took a photo of the alpaca that wee James was leading around the alpaca farm near Stirling. The bright sunlit whiteness of its head contrasted beautifully with the dark storm clouds in the distance. I was delighted; a fab thing to put up on Facebook when I got home!

Wendy had been organising lots of things to do during our holidays now that our visit to Disneyland was cancelled, due to the pandemic. Those holidays were so needed. I had already extended them because I had been getting very irritable at work: being more challenging in response to innocent emails than I had ever been before, less able to complete pieces of work to my satisfaction. My boss had given me her blessing to take leave at short notice; it was a great relief. I had thought it would solve everything.

I was also delighted for another reason. Wendy had got me to talk the night before, and I had confessed that I still couldn't go back to work at the end of my holidays. Somehow it was like I had run full tilt into a brick wall and was stumbling around, dazed, no longer knowing what direction I was facing. I didn't know what to do. I was contemplating resigning and trying to work out how we could all manage on Wendy's part-time wages or whether I could get any benefits. I wanted to take time off sick but didn't think not being able to work was a good enough reason. After all, I could cook meals, wash the clothes, talk, laugh, and walk Dash the dog. I could more or less function. Wendy told me to speak to my CPN. My boss told me to speak to my CPN.

I do not know what caused this sudden shift for me. Maybe, as with lots of people, it was the stress of the pandemic. I know I was finding facilitating, and taking notes of Zoom calls with people I had never met before, increasingly tiring. I also know that I could no longer laugh off the frequent harassment I had been getting for over a year from a few people who were very angry at me about what I do in the world of mental health. It may have been as simple as the fact that a year ago, almost to the day, my dad had died while I was on holiday and I still had not shed a tear or talked about it that much.

Whatever it was, I went for my fortnightly injection with my CPN, and she immediately told me there would be no problem with taking sick leave, that I needed to speak with my GP.

Later, just as we were queueing to go up Dumbarton Rock, my phone rang. After less than thirty seconds speaking to a GP I had never met before, I was signed off sick for a month. After all, I think there are some advantages to having a diagnosis of schizophrenia and being on a Compulsory Treatment Order.

For me, this signified a massive shift in my thinking and way of living. I was incredibly proud that despite my diagnosis and hospital admissions, I was managing seven staff at one point, that I had never used up my sick leave entitlement. It pains me now to say it, but my approach to work has been very unhealthy. I immerse myself in it fully. I can be so consumed by what I am doing that I pay no attention to life outside of my laptop. Until now, I have never voluntarily taken time off because of mental illness. I have worked right up to the point that I am sectioned and taken off to constant observation in hospital. When I am discharged, I always go back to work within days of getting home. It absorbs me at the expense of things that are far more important, such as the people I love in my life.

Furthermore, now I was taking sick leave just because I couldn't face work… It didn't make sense to me. I felt incredibly guilty, and out of that guilt, I made some critical decisions.

I have a close colleague from the past who told me she took time off when she was depressed and was reported to her workplace when she was seen outside, walking in the street. I have a friend who I sometimes go walking with when she is off sick. She knows I am always posting on Facebook and always tells me not to post pictures of her looking happy. She says some people cannot be trusted and she could be in huge trouble if seen out enjoying herself when she is meant to be ill. I find that confusing.

It seems such a short-sighted way of dealing with life and such things as mental illness. I knew full well that the worst thing I could do would be to lose myself in my thoughts, and let those thoughts I try to avoid gain power when I was feeling vulnerable. The very worst thing to do would be to stop and isolate myself, as I was very tempted to do.

I told my boss that I would be doing everything I could to enjoy myself while I was off sick: giving myself treats, going out, as far as the restrictions permitted, posting photos of me being happy, laughing, looking carefree.

To my delight, my boss said, "Please do, take a break. Do what you need to do to get well again. Only come back when you can face work again and are well." And so, I did.

I think my favourite times were walking Dash the dog. We have many places we go, but I love Ardmore Point, a couple of miles from our house. Dash loves it too. He goes wild in the back of the car when he realises we are about to turn down the small road to the edge of the Firth. We walk. I look at the geese in the field, take photos of my favourite solitary tree; listen to the curlews and oystercatchers, watch the lumpy flight of the herons, the sudden swirl of water where a seal has been peering at us.

The number of times Wendy took me to the café in the square in Helensburgh… I ate so many heart-attack-inducing cheese toasties, and wittered to the wonderful waiting staff who always came up to give Dash the dog treats and water where we sat talking, in the gazebo that they had erected for Covid.

I posted on social media when wee Charlotte gave me great big hugs and said she loved me and when James managed to look up from his Xbox and say, "Thank you," when I took his tea to his room.

As I write this, three and half months later, I am contemplating starting work again; only half a day to start with, but I can face it now. I can relish the fact that work has said I can now block some of the people who send the most abusive emails, if they carry on sending them. I have agreed to stop making my days when I am working so intense that it takes me ages to get back to the real world when I finish at the end of the day.

I can also remember those Zoom calls I cancelled where my peers said, "Of course you should cancel, you need to look after yourself." Furthermore, this time, I will really take what they say to heart.

I remember Wendy saying she was very proud of me because I had taken responsibility for my mental health for the first time in almost ever, and avoided one of those admissions I hate so much. Because, of course, those realities I hate did sometimes overtake me. I did worry that I was destroying the world; that I was responsible for Covid, Syria, global warming. I did email the church to ask them, although I was a devil and an atheist, could I come to their church for sanctuary? I tried to get my CPN to understand that I was ruining my family's life and needed to leave them but felt trapped because that would also ruin their life, and so couldn't leave.

I have had a chance to relax, get up late, listen to the radio and music; to tell work I was doing all I could to enjoy myself. To witter about all the things I was up to on social media and receive a consistently supportive response to that.

Isn't that how life should be?

I paint a rosy picture. It isn't quite like that, really. I still feel guilty for taking time off sick, my frequent trips to cheer me up didn't always cheer me up. Sometimes, if I was alone on my walks in the hills and by the shore, thoughts I had hoped to avoid overtook me. My refuge in my room upstairs sometimes wasn't that at all. Instead, it was a place to stare at the ceiling, not listening to the radio and remembering things I don't want to remember. I did still worry about the reaction I might get if I was too cheerful on Facebook.

Is it still possible that when people are off sick because of poor mental health, they feel they need to look sad, miserable and exhausted?

Never leave the house, do nothing at all for fear of being seen as frauds and malingerers?

I think it is. I must admit I still feel guilty at my walk with my sister in Arrochar and our meal at the Village Inn. Indeed, if I could drive there and talk away, I could also log onto my emails, attend Zoom meetings and write reports… But, of course, I couldn't. I need to understand that I still subject myself to all the stereotypes of what poor mental health looks like and how we need to deal with it. However, finally, it seems I have made a start, and my workplace has made sure that coming back to work will hopefully be the best start in a long time.

2021—JANUARY—SANDY—THAT LULL BETWEEN DIFFERENT WARS, THE ONE THAT NEVER QUITE GOES AWAY: INTRODUCING YOU TO SANDY AND HIS FAMILY.

I first met Sandy, Wendy's dad, not long after I came down to live with Wendy in Cardross, way back in late 2015.

I will not be the person who tells you too many details of Sandy's life, in case you are hoping for that. I was just witness to Sandy's last few years when he had already been diagnosed with terminal prostate cancer.

I got to know him very well in those years, but I am not particularly curious and have neither the questions in my head nor the memory to remember the details of his life. I do remember him playing football with James. I remember him laughing and slumped, exhausted. I remember his belief that family was more important than anything else. I remember he was lovely and maybe that is all I need to remember. That he was not only lovely, but he loved those around him and sought out ways to make them happier in their lives. It is all I need really, the smile when he saw us at the door; the beginning of conversation already.

I still don't quite know what he did when he was working. I know he worked for the council and was something to do with chartered surveying.

He had wanted to be a pilot but was colour blind so that never happened. He studied geology at university but never completed the course because one of his parents got ill. I think that was it. He told me so many things, so many times, but I have forgotten most of them. It seems wrong somehow. A betrayal of him.

He told us lots of stories about his work, but they were mainly about driving days, like trying to get round Islay and Jura and back home to Balloch in one day, or the time he outran a police car which was chasing him for speeding when he was driving from England to Scotland, and didn't he have a crash somewhere down there too? I think he did. He said he was a very safe driver but I have a memory of too many stories of bashed-in cars. I remember he also talked of doing some free surveying for some good cause which he was proud about and that he hated it when he was sent to Mull or Oban, and how I would tease him about that because, unlike him, I think both places are lovely.

There were also tales about his anger at some of the politicians he was answerable to, some of the corruption he witnessed. More often, he would talk about cricket matches and football games and the ancestor who played for Hibs. He talked about judo with Peter, about Wendy at dance class when they were young and again, the different cars he had.

Wendy and I would groan (me, inaudibly) when he went on to the technical details of some long gone car from the past and what went wrong with it and what it did. But still he talked of them and still I listened and still they both said, with a laugh, that I was very polite; maybe too polite…

We did the same with his tales of military history. I have never seen a house with so many books about wars and the machines that make wars; walls and walls of books, box after box and shelf after shelf of magazines, reference cards; four different computers cross referencing his years and years of research. All those years and yet, when he sought libraries or organisations that might want access to the materials after he died, no one had any interest. That must have been such a hard thing for him to hear.

He spent ages trying to find records of the Fighter Squadron my dad had been a pilot in, printed off pictures of Lightnings, passed over special editions of aviation magazines which featured the aircraft my dad flew.

Sandy married his childhood friend, Janet. She was the only girlfriend he ever had. When Wendy tells me of her childhood, she talks of it with a great deal of affection. She says she was always loved and she always knew she was and that that is by far the most important thing. That she was always out doing things. Every evening she would be either dancing or with the horses, or she might be doing amateur dramatics or music or, on the weekends in the summer, spending hours, very bored, watching her dad at his cricket matches. She tells me that she experienced considerable joy as she was growing up, that she was good, though shy in class but that sometimes there was some great mischievousness.

Like the time she and her friend were chucked out of Balloch Tourist Office because they constantly went in pretending to be French schoolgirls with very little English and very strong French accents, or the fun they had throwing wire under the wheels of passing cars because it made them skid in such a funny way, or how they liked replying with insults to the man in the flats who was always phoning the public phone box, asking young girls to come to his flat, and how they giggled when they phoned boys at the local public school and made dates to meet them which they never kept. Or the brick she threw at the boy she hated which she thought would never hit him but did.

How she always lost her house key and had to wait in the garden for her parents to get home from work which didn't help when she was desperate for a wee.

Or the time when she and her brother (Peter) had wound her mum up so much that she shouted at them that she didn't want another squeak out of them and how Wendy couldn't resist going, "Eeek!" only to be dragged out of the sitting room by her hair.

She stayed at home when she went to university and went out partying most nights. Last night she told me she partied for about fifteen years, found it hard to understand that I was settled in a relationship at twenty-four with a baby at twenty-eight, that at that age she still had another ten years of partying in front of her.

When she was at home, earlier in her life, she said she would wake bleary-eyed in the morning, and her mum would often tap on the door to her bedroom with a fried breakfast for her. She loved that.

Or those times Peter played that game with her where you throw knives between your feet and she was terrified. Or when, for some weird reason, she and a friend made a fire on the sitting room carpet and seeing the molten mess they had created, she rearranged the sitting room so the couch was over the burn mark. How, for ages after, she did all the cleaning in that room in the hope that the damage would never be seen.

I remember her talking about her first primary school, which she loved, and how upset she was that she went to a different school when her Nana died. How, to start with, she had few friends but quickly made new ones though some of the friends of these new friends resented her for it.

I find it strange to think that Wendy has such a longstanding circle of friends; people she partied with in her late teens and in her twenties, she still knows, still parties with. These friends, some of whom she knew even earlier, when they were just children.

She has seen them get jobs, fall in and out of love, get ill, recover and sometimes not, have children, get divorced, find new partners, move away and always come back. I don't understand this at all.

I know almost no one from my twenties, let alone my teens. To witness and share your childhood, to get old with people who have lived only a few miles from you for most of your life. What on earth would that be like? I think it would be wonderful; that knowledge, that sense of connection and understanding and belonging. I am jealous, I think. I like that Wendy's friends are opinionated and keen to share their opinions, that they are open and have experienced many of the harder elements of being alive but remain loving and both strong and vulnerable.

I love the story of how once, on the train, her girlfriends removed some very aggressive and drunk men from it without even pausing to wonder if that was wise. They are not bound by the caution I have cultivated for so long, always conscious of the words that should and shouldn't be used; the beliefs and values that you really must have to fit in in my tiny, tiny circle. Their presence is liberating. The generosity of the living of their lives, and the sharing of their experiences and their food, and just their presence, is wonderful. And all those stories of different nightclubs and escapades that would not be accepted nowadays. Like when a group of them went out selling kisses in the pubs for a pound a kiss, to raise money for meningitis research after one of them fell ill with it and recovered, and how they raised a fair few hundred pounds. Between them they have a library of stories filled with laughter, tears, adventures that would make the average soap opera seem dull and uneventful.

A supportive band of women, growing up together, sharing the worst of life and the best of life, always there for each other, able to laugh and be silly but also to dwell in the dark on the things we all go through. I cannot imagine what it would be like to know that I could have a set of friends who I know will always be in my life, how could you even dream of such things?

Living in 'the Vale', some people assume you must have a pretty grim upbringing, but Wendy lived in nice houses and areas, her family was never really short of money. She tended to be well behaved with only the slightest of naughty traits. She tells me she was shy and hardly talked at school but that she was very popular. She tells me that she was insecure when she reached adulthood and would have seemed very aloof.

She tells me that, even now, she is very shy and that she prefers not to be with other people. I find that remarkable because, whenever she is in company she always talks. She both entertains and listens; she can be caring or, in the right company, crude, funny and slightly outrageous.

She says this is exhausting but that there is a need to communicate when you are in a place where that is expected. I find that alien. 'How on earth can you do that?' I think to myself, while she looks at me, when I seem to be happily at ease in company, saying nothing at all; smiling a lot but not speaking, sometimes threatening to take a book with me to gatherings, though luckily it is some years since I last did that. I think the lack of effort I appear to make horrifies her, and my statements that I usually have nothing to say, nothing even resting somewhere in my head, bemuse her.

She does remember how her dad could have something of an anger in him, that she and Peter would try not to look at him when he was in one of his moods. She also remembers that Christmas was often not so good as her dad was determined to do all the cooking and get it just right and how, by having to make it perfect, it rarely was; especially when they were older and sitting down to dinner with hangovers.

She remembers her mum's bad driving, how she was, and still is, a genius with numbers, worked in a bank, a kitchen showroom and a bookies. She tells me of the amazing cakes her mum got her for her birthdays, how life with her family was so good.

Wendy tells me how her gran would take Peter home for lunch when he was at school and yet she had to go to the shops for her lunch, but that she has such fond memories of the shop she went to. The one that had the machine which would slice a piece of meat for her sandwich. She describes the sound of the clean slice of that circling disc and brings it to life in my own different memories. She tells me one of her grans died of cirrhosis and that, although she drank, she never seemed drunk, that she seemed to drink to cope with her anxiety. And she says the other gran came to live in their house when she was dying and that the death of both her parents' mums scarred her parents deeply.

She says that Sandy, witnessing his mum's long, long, drawn out pain, and having felt that pain for so many months, did not want anyone in his family to have to go through such a thing with him. And how her mum, with her own countless visits to hospital in the past, grew to absolutely loathe the thought of ever going through the doors of such places ever again.

Her dad did a bit of a family tree which showed that his side of the family had lived in the area for hundreds of years. He got back as far as 1745 in Cardross, but then, over in Luss, there are graves of McAuslans that go back even further. They moved between Bonhill, Jamestown and Alexandria, with a brief diversion to Glasgow.

He talked about growing up in Dumbarton. Now what did his dad do? How annoying! He told me so many times and now I can't remember. Was it to do with accounts? And wasn't there someone who collected insurance and spent lots of time on the golf course? And wasn't his dad not so good to him, now I think of it? Back to the anger and the alcohol again, maybe? Which maybe explains why Sandy almost never drank.

Wendy's mum is very unique and sometimes Wendy doesn't believe all the things she tells her but I remember, one birthday, Wendy researched some of her mum's English roots and found out that one of her ancestors was indeed described as a Gentleman in the census, and that he owned a very smart pub and that when his wife died, he married the chambermaid and had more children with her. She printed off a photo she found of the pub and the people, and contacted the pub.

I think for a time Wendy had plans to take her mum down to England to see it but, as can happen, that didn't occur.

Despite being married for many, many years and having been childhood sweethearts, Wendy's dad and her mum grew apart and when Wendy had grown up, they split up. They never formally divorced and lived near each other afterwards.

Sandy kept on visiting Janet, doing odds and ends for her, right up until his last nine months or so when that became too much for him.

Wendy told me how she had been telling Sandy for years to go to see the doctor about his need to wee all the time and yet I remember, not long before his death, he was saying how important it was to get checked out and said there had been no signs or symptoms of his illness to pick up on before it had become too late.

It is much easier to think we could have done nothing about something like that than to think, *if only I had gone to the doctor.* I do the same. I still have packages to test myself for bowel cancer but haven't done it. I routinely think I am dying of something or other, and even when I think it seriously instead of half-heartedly, I never go along to the doctor. It is really stupid but I think I just don't want to encourage illness by asking for it to be checked out.

Even though I have witnessed Sandy's journey to death and I am going to write some of it down, I do not think I will come up with anything hugely profound or new on the subject of either the living I have started doing with Wendy's family, or the dying that Sandy and my dad had to prepare for, but maybe the very mundanity of things such as this, the things that struck me and which I learned from, will bring something to some of you reading this.

February

2021—FEBRUARY—WENDY—SATURDAY SHAPE-SHIFTING

"That ceiling is so white! I like white rooms! I like the lightshade, how it is like a waterfall of silver," said Wendy later, while lying beside me.

Waking on a morning without the children, slow stretch to the edges of the bed, bleary-eyed gaze into the darkness, the edges of the room lighting up with the bright winter sun behind the windowshades.

Dash on his back – legs splayed apart, paws dangling in front of his muzzle like some rag dog, an occasional whimper but whether it is a whimper of pleasure or not, I do not know.

I am so bored of Radio 4. All the news and news and news. I would prefer to listen to my own homegrown family news: what Charlotte was whispering about to her mum last night, how the rabbits are faring, when the decking will finally be replaced.

I am hot and sweaty after my sleep and the warmth of the room from the heating in the morning.

Lying half-dreaming, I cannot pause my life for the dawning of inspiration but, just listen to those geese flying overhead! Remember the sound of the owls from last night and think of the rooks bustling, getting ready for spring to start.

In the shower, the grime, the harsh thoughts of last night wash away. I feel warmed and cleansed, my mind loses its fuzzy sleep, small prickles of shampoo scratch at my closed eyes and all around I feel warm water, the splash of a bright day which I can take my time to join. This is bliss and my heavy, heavy towel is a strange sort of bliss too.

Clambering back into bed, Dash is in a different place, not too inclined to begin the day either. I am just slightly damp, but feeling so soft, so clean, so fresh; such a wonderful feeling to lie back in bed on clean sheets with nothing to get up for.

I can hear the tread of Wendy on the stairs and grin, pretending to stare at Facebook. She creeps into the room with a greeting and bundled up in a downie, slides into bed besides me; tells me I smell nice, snuggles up for kisses, caresses. I love our caresses, I love it when the downie falls away from her and she reaches for me.

The rooks are still making a noise, the blackbird is singing an alarm call, there is the sound of a car outside, a person calling to their dog.

Wendy tells me to close the window, to seal in the day, turns on the light beside me and spends the next half hour making hand shadows on the ceiling. The ducks and dogs and monsters all have names and stories; all those stories I will forget, the crudeness they get up to, the silliness they embark on. They flutter across the ceiling while Wendy's bare arms weave above our faces in the morning air.

I am entranced, spend my time giggling.

"You are so silly!" I say.

"You have a go," you say and I refuse for as long as I can until you ask incredulously, "What is that?" to the shape I make on the wall. And I have no idea. I giggle even more.

"I don't know, I can't do things like this," I say.

You lean over and kiss me, your hand lingers. We lie back and stare at the ceiling, the bright clean white room and our multicoloured bedsheets. We start to plan a makeover, decide against it, breakfast waits on us. We are in no hurry.

These moments where you do not have to move, achieve, don't have to do anything but giggle at shapes on the ceiling. If there is no word for this feeling, no philosophical entry to describe the bliss of lying side by side with your hearts wide to the world, if there are no words and no theories, I had better invent them.

This month started off with frost, cold biting wind and then snow, turned in the end to almost spring-like temperatures.

We juggled the home-schooling and work. I sat in my eyrie, high in the house, in the small gap where the dormer window sits. I can see the pond we made out of the guinea pig cage. It is full of watercress and every day when I look over the top of my laptop, I will, at some point, see the magpies washing in the water.

It is hardest for Wendy, I think, trying to work her extra hours, deal with the crises at work and at the same time deal with the children. But the children struggle too. They miss their friends so much and, although James will talk to people on his Xbox, and Charlotte to her friends on Zoom, it is not the same as that everyday contact. Wendy and I think their teacher is pretty fab. She puts so much into her classes but the children are growing to dislike her, mainly because when she asks them what they would like to do, she ignores their choices and goes with her own preferences. They are slowly beginning to hate the Gaelic lessons she likes to give them and their French lessons. Actually, they are slowly beginning to hate all things school-based except the thought of one day playing with their friends again.

At my CTO meeting I asked my psychiatrist about the person who appears in front of me when I think of Wendy. You know when you are having a conversation in your mind with someone you love, or wondering about something or other connected to them? When I do that, for a moment I get a glimpse of a person staring at me, commenting on me in a horrible way, judging me, staring at me with her pale expression, her dark eyes and hair. It distracts me from the wonder of my present life, makes me uneasy and frightened. It damages how I see Wendy; this person interfering with our life.

I think this image has something to do with my ex-wife and wish so much she wasn't there. The psychiatrist talked about avatar therapy, but then backtracked when I said I couldn't actually hear what she was saying. Wendy thought she was an intrusive thought born of trauma. I think she has nothing to with schizophrenia and tend to agree with Wendy. My CPN says hallucinations come in many forms and that confuses me. It also makes me think that none of the things I have asked for in my tribunals have ever come to be; that the famous principle of reciprocity is a farce, that people really are content to leave us be because they have no expectation that change will happen or impetus to try to help us make it happen.

Despite the wonder of my new life, I still keep too busy and make life a series of achievements and tasks, even if they are just about cooking and shopping, or writing speeches and books. It helps me hide from my constant thoughts of death and all the despair that accompanies such feelings. They are so old that I doubt I know how to ever escape from that way of being.

But at the same time I can also see how I feel the opposite.

I do think I shut down for almost a year after first moving in to Wendy's house. I had been used to doing my own thing and for everything I did to be more or less what I wanted to do. I had been used to sitting at the end of the harbour wall at sunset and walking the beach whenever I wanted. I had a very busy and consuming work life. I had a collection of friends I was always seeing and suddenly I was in a house where life was busy; where there were dirty plates everywhere and discarded clothes on every surface.

I found two very dramatic children in my life, one of whom seemed very suspicious of me, who kept saying he wanted his mummy and daddy to live in the same house. He is lovely, popular, funny, wry, quiet in company and in front of his teachers but so talkative with his friends and mum. He is already cleverer than I will ever be but maybe he looks askance at me for my inability to get over that initial suspicion.

Though we still fancied each other, it wasn't the first thing on our minds when we walked into the house. We were more consumed with dying dads, or the pain and exhaustion Wendy's endometriosis was causing her, or the politics of work or my long hours on the days I had to go to Edinburgh or off to Inverness, Aberdeen, Dumfries.

And we both had, or have, such needs. Me? I want to be constantly praised and adored, and Wendy? I think she would just love to have conversations and some spontaneity and please, please, no more organising, no more working out what to do or buy; no more lists, no more dates to put in diaries. I think she and I would like to go back to the time when we couldn't stop talking and when I always had ideas of who to see and things to do; so much to do that Wendy would plead for a break and time just for ourselves, to ourselves.

More likely she would have liked just to have gone back to the time when her dad was well and her mum still let me in her house; when all this sadness just wasn't happening.

And so I can see why I might still have those days when I am alone, wandering around wanting to die; it is hardly as if depression and schizophrenia just drop away with a change in lifestyle.

After moving down to my new family, I feel I somehow lost any spontaneity, my voice and the lightness I had at last gained in those first years of dating. I don't know, it is so long since I have been free of that blankness in me, that lack of life. Did I regain it when we were wandering the beaches, impatient for kisses? Or is it always there, has it always been there? In many ways I thought that confirmed how evil I was. I thought I saw the effect of my behaviour on my new family and hated it. I felt trapped; yearning for death and yet yearning for this blessed life at the same time. Worried about those thoughts I don't share in real life, terrified about what would happen if it all went wrong again and I subjected Wendy and the children to that mat of darkness that occupies my soul. And yet Wendy says I am the most gentle and loving person she knows and I cannot understand this.

I look at the things that have happened to our families and think this is more evidence that I am evil. That finally I have proof that I am a devil. And so often I want to act on this, or if not act on it, up sticks, leave Wendy and the children so they can have someone better in their lives.

At such times I feel trapped, but then I think of how awful it would be for our family if I were dead or damaged or in hospital and how I have to protect them from my darker thoughts and actions.

When I found out Sandy was dying, not that long after meeting him for the first time, I found myself reminded about how much I have sought death and I found myself slightly aghast. Sandy wanted every precious moment he could have, delighting in his family and yet I, who hope to be a fundamental part of the fabric of this family, this new life, live only a few sentences in my mind from the need to die. I look at the arrogance that I have which means that with each new tribulation we experience I see new evidence that I do not belong here; that I am the cause of the unhappiness that everyone has gone through over the last few years. That here is evidence that, far from the randomness of life, I have been steering those I love down some path to mutual tragedy.

Let me peer back. Back to this death thing. When I was little, death was not a concept I understood in any way. It was as alien as the idea that the squiggles that my mum put on paper were actually words and yet at some point, the dots joined and just as I had the delighted revelation about what writing was, so did I have that terror in the pit of the stomach when one day I realised I would actually die.

I think it would have been when Dad was working in High Wycombe with Fighter Command and we lived in a small, very modern house, in a cul de sac, surrounded by young families with children our age, just in our first years of school.

Richard (my brother) and I shared a room and I remember leaping into my bed, frightened that monsters would get me. I would snuggle right under the covers, pulling them right over my head, wedging the pillow to make a small place for the air to get in. And there I would lie, worried about those monsters; also worried about dying, worrying that I would not wake up in the morning.

That abyss that I thought about occurred to me throughout my childhood and it terrified me.

I think it was initially that white terror, that sick feeling that I would not *be* one day which was later added to when I became a fervent Evangelical Christian, when I was at prep school, terrified that I would go to hell.

Although I wanted to be saved, I didn't think I was. I had never spoken in tongues, could not feel that ecstasy at finding Jesus in my heart. I desperately wanted to. I went to Scripture Union, dreamed of becoming a missionary but no, to tell the truth, I did not reach the mark. I thought when I died, I was doomed to unbearable suffering for ever and ever and was so frightened.

Later, in characteristic fashion, I became a fundamentalist atheist and sought out the Christians at university to tell them how silly religion was. I was also shocked and upset by death, telling them there was no point in life, no God, no anything really.

I thought to myself that if there is no God then there is no meaning, no purpose, no point to anything. It horrified me.

I spent many drunken hours thinking of the lack of meaning, thinking perversely that if there is no point and meaning, then death would be a better option. I grasped at Nietzsche and Camus and Sartre but I never understood them.

I think it was those lonely days, trying to make sense of the world and trying to make sense of *me*, that terrible self-consciousness that manifested itself in wearing raggedy clothes, speaking in a whisper, speaking in a foreign accent I shouldn't have had, walking out of lecture theatres to the derisive comments of the lecturer, but driven by panic.

Those times. Going blank at the ticket counter of a train station, not being able to buy the ticket or articulate what I was feeling.

That terrible time when I hated my parents, had no friends, was desperate for a girlfriend but thought I must be gay as I was so shy I found it almost impossible to talk to girls.

Ah! That morass of growing up that I couldn't manage, which I translated as a principled hatred of life, a principled philosophical wish to die, when all I was, was just plain old frightened and upset by life and becoming an adult. And terribly, terribly lonely.

And now, when I think of my evil, I assume I will suffer hugely when I die but sometimes I feel I have been forgiven for being a devil. And sometimes I fall back into that atheism I somehow have and, despite being convinced of my evil, think, in the absence of imminent death, that when I die it might be quite good.

I love to sleep. I really, really, love oblivion. The thought of just drifting into that nothingness that is death, feels peaceful and comfortable: pain free, soft. It would be so good not to have to think or worry or feel sadness or despair. Or at least that is what I tell myself.

But I think that is an intellectual understanding because when I am in that place in my world where I think I might be dying (I have decided I have toe cancer at the moment), at these points, I panic. I think how desperately sad I would be not to see the trees, hear the sea and the birdsong, not to have a whisky at the bench in the garden in the evening sun. Not to be able to walk hand in hand with Wendy while the children chatter and run around the walled garden with all its flowers and colours at Geilston, see the green haze, the grass and plants by its tiny burn.

Not to see and be part of all that, would be so terribly, terribly sad. I could not bear that.

I told you that I would provide no answers, give no truths. I just paint a slight picture of my mind, my life and slight, slight sketches of the people around me. I would that I could do more.

Sandy made these thoughts more real but also gave me a perspective on issues and ideas I had never really confronted before in any meaningful way. He presented me with the reality of what dying is really like. He also, over the years, took away some of the abject terror I have felt for so many years about death.

I cannot imagine how Sandy felt over those years when he knew he was going to die soon. I know that some of his nights were dark, that he did not sleep; that he worried and pondered and also felt the intense physical pain his illness was causing. That must have been a constant reminder he couldn't escape from.

I think he was very brave indeed. I think in some ways he eased our minds with the positivity that he nurtured so much. There were times, later, when he truly struggled and Wendy, confronted by that struggle, suffered greatly, but for so much of the time they just managed.

It may be trite and silly to talk about putting a brave face on things, but I think everyone's collective determination to do so made some of the darkest of moods more fleeting, less intense. I know in the last few years I learnt an incredible amount, from both Sandy and my dad, and from Wendy and her family and friends. And now that I think about it, I can so easily see why fairy stories just can't be the fairy stories they should be. That the dynamic and marvellous family life I now have really is a fairy story come true. I believe that to my core.

But, in fairy stories we do not have to remember to empty the bins or buy light bulbs and we do not need to learn to be sensitive to the needs of confused and bewildered children and present to help with the grief and exhaustion of our fairy princess. Somehow the complexity of emotion seems left for the villains, but I am sure that fairy princesses get tired and can feel bitter and find they want to sleep all the time and that fairy princes are insecure and uncertain and incapable of navigating the high and random emotion of young and fractious children.

But those fairy stories have a power. I still yearn for my fairy story. I think I feel resentment when the leftover food falls out of the bag in the food waste bin and I have to scrape it back in; annoyance that the shed stank so much when a hedgehog sought refuge there in the winter and died there and I had to scrape the remains away; frustration that I have to have Dash the dog on the lead so much because he wants to run far away, chasing deer. Why can't he be like a normal dog and come when I ask him to? And why wasn't I able to teach him to? None of this feels very prince-like and I find I am not happy with that at all. Wow. I never knew these were some of my expectations! Where on earth did this all spring from?

When I think of these things, I find myself confused. Today, Wendy was asking me about how I make sense of things and understand how I am feeling and I had to reply that I rarely know. It takes ages and ages for anything to make sense to me or to connect. My dad being dead and appearing in my dreams? Is this a resolution? I don't think I will ever really, totally believe he is dead. Sandy's journey in the years I knew him, it fades a little nowadays. I forget the wonderful things he did to make the children feel good, to laugh with the family. I am really stuck on that getting on with it thing, and much as I hate to say it, that stiff upper lip thing.

I think I need to come to terms with some of the things that happened to me, because they have a power to ruin the relationships I have in my life. But also, I am not sure that it is always good to talk, or always good to live by feeling and emotion. Sometimes, when subject to things that are unbearable, you need to shut down a little, avoid the tears, steel your heart and manage to get up every day, again and again, even when you doubt you are capable of it.

It is maybe a quaint and unfashionable thought that young people would look at askance, that the setters of opinion would frown about, but I find when I consider the effect I have on others because of how I feel, or when I let myself fall maudlin with memory or emotion at the end of the evening, it rarely helps me and certainly doesn't help those around me. In some ways I am keen not to acknowledge how I feel, perhaps because I just don't know how I feel, or perhaps because I cannot deal with it if I face it.

It is strange to write these words and to think that people might use them to show how damaged a certain generation was because of how it was expected to deal with life, its ups and downs and in-betweens.

This month I have written speeches about peer research, another one on the involvement of people like me in the Scott Review and another about how services should respond to people in crisis. It is so much harder to do them on a video platform. I print them off and peer slightly to the side of the computer where I read them, propped on the book stand I was given after a visit to Zaragoza for work, many years ago.

The Scott Review – I joined that a year ago as a member of the five person executive and last December was made joint vice chair along with Karen (a carer). It is such an ambitious project. We are reviewing all the strands of mental health legislation in the context of a United Nations Committee that says it is discriminatory. We are also looking at all the other rights that apply to us – our social, economic and cultural rights, and we have been doing it in the middle of Covid with a much smaller secretariat than we need. I find it quite terrifying, to be honest.

Anyway, the audience in my talk about the Scott Review… There were a couple of people who detest me at work. I don't know if they still send out abusive tweets and emails, because I have finally been allowed to block them and the Scott Review has also told them that their behaviour is not welcome and nor are they.

It is a big step to silence anyone and to be honest, they are not silenced; they pop up all over the place with their abuse. I found out they were likely to be present at the university webinar where I was speaking and found myself hollow in my stomach. I just did not want to see them listening to me or hear them questioning me or even view them in the chat. I asked the university to stop them attending and the organisers tried their best but I suppose the controversy over 'no platforming' can work against things like this. One of my abusers came to the conference but chat was private and monitored. I saw him though, felt that sick dread they have provoked recently. It is funny that people claiming to be human rights activists, who deny that they have ever experienced mental illness or even been carers, are able to drive people to distraction who know all too well the sadness of illness and spend late nights worrying if they will be able to do that public speech. My speech went ok on the day but I still think it is wrong.

Despite February being the month of my birthday – and it was such a wonderful birthday – it is also a month of harsh memories. It is the month in which my tribunals are held every two years and I get sectioned again and again, to my complete relief and abject despair. It is the month that I finally stopped my payments to my son, four years ago, and felt some shame that when I worked out if the days I have seen him since I left my wife were worked out as a proportion of payment, that I would have paid seven and half thousand pounds for each day I have seen him, and of course that is not the point, but it adds to my sadness. And finally, it is the month that Sandy's journey since I came here five years ago came to its end, one of the most powerful and intense events I have ever experienced and one I hope not to experience again.

2021—FEBRUARY—ALAN—AN INTRODUCTION

My dad had a strange childhood. We did not talk much about such things in the family, really. I think mainly because he was a little confused by it but also, somehow, we are not a family that tells stories. I think I learnt more about my mum in the gap between lockdowns when Charlotte sat with us at the table and quizzed her for hours on her childhood, than I had ever known. And what I know of my dad, I am mainly learning from his memoir, which I am slowly reading, more than a year after his death.

My dad's dad, Harold, was Welsh, brought up in a huge house in Maesycwmmer with tennis courts, outbuildings and a chapel. Something or other happened and he went to London with one of his brothers and I don't think he talked to his family again. They owned a fish and chip shop in the East End. That is where he met and married Clarice Evans. Her dad was a carpenter; she was born and bred in the East of London but went to the same church as him which is where they met.

Just reading his memoir makes me confused. I am so far from that life. My ancestors feel completely alien to me. I have no connection to them at all. It is interesting to me but even their names and the places they lived bear no relation to my reality.

My dad was born in Ilford on 8 April 1937. I found this extract from his memoir which I find startling in its contrast to my own upbringing:

My earliest memory was the bombing of London Docks in 1940. I would have been three. My father took me into the garden one night. It was dark, but the sky was red, bright almost as daylight as the warehouses burnt... Houses in London were issued with shelters. We had an indoor shelter... which had a heavy steel top, substantial steel corner girders and heavy duty wire netting between the girders. This was in the living room and acted as a table. We ate and slept in or on the shelter.

When the Blitz started, it was not good to live in London and my mother and I went to stay with Grandmother Morgan (known as Nan) in Hengoed, Glamorgan. Her house was 'Cartref', the end house in Chapel Terrace. It must have been relatively spacious since in addition to us and Nan, Marjory (Uncle Edwin's wife) also abandoned London and stayed in 'Cartref' with several of her family, plus I think Dilys and her friend Alice Cherry were there. My memories of Nan were of a Welsh version of the older Queen Victoria – short, dumpy and dressed in black: formidable... I remember the house as being strict. Welsh Baptists are unrelentingly religious. Every Sunday meant Chapel, morning and evening plus Sunday School... Only religious books were allowed on Sunday. Newspapers or magazines were banned and radio severely restricted.

I started school in Hengoed, walking with my cousins across the 'Grieg', heathland above the valley. I remember the sound of the wind whistling through the telephone lines. I survived, surprisingly, as a sickly and cosseted English kid turning up in a Welsh mining village. I do not remember much bullying. Discipline was strict, a ruler across the knuckles was the usual punishment for talking in class... Back to the sickly. I did have asthma. Many times I was hunched with a towel over my head over a bowl of hot water with Friars Balsam. My mother said I had a 'weak chest', so was only allowed out with scarf, pullovers and coat. My cousin Ruth was staying in Hengoed at the same time, she said she can only remember once when I was allowed out to run and play on the Grieg with my cousins like any young boy should.

My mother and grandmother did not get on – to put it mildly. Whether she felt out of place, coming from a working class East End family and living with what had been a reasonably wealthy middle class Welsh family, or whether she just was not prepared to make the effort to fit in, I do not know. What I do know is that as soon as the bombing in London had reduced, she dragged me back with her to live with her sister Grace in East London. Then the V-1s started. These were pilotless aircraft with

42

a couple of thousand pounds of high explosive. They had a distinctive pulse jet engine, it throbbed. All was well while you could hear the engine, but when it stopped you knew that the V-1 was now gliding and in a minute or so, would hit and explode. The silence was terrifying. Almost as terrifying was the sound of the AA guns and especially the rocket batteries which were on Wanstead Flats. V-1s hit houses in the street where we were living and the next street. V-2s then came along. These rockets were supersonic and as such were rather less scary, since you did not hear them coming. First came the explosion. If you heard it, you were alive. I cannot remember going to school during this time, I have no idea what we did during the days. I believe we went back to Wales for a time before returning to London and back to Falmouth Gardens for VE Day.

My mum has a similar story of war, and talks of living in Teignmouth, of air raids and ornaments falling from the walls with the blast of explosions. She cannot remember how long she and her baby sister spent as evacuees in rural Devon but did not seem to have seen her mum for months at a time. Her dad was on the Russian convoys and her mum ran a guest house or hotel. A memory that sticks with me is that when she came back home, she never had a bedroom of her own, that she would just sleep in whatever room was not being used for guests. I wonder at how little I remember of my parent's stories. I find them fascinating but forget most of the facts after each telling.

I do remember that my dad's parents were very religious but the strength of it never really affected or influenced us. When we visited them in Devon, where my dad's parents had settled after the war, they would sometimes take us to church. I vaguely remember long, long incomprehensible services. I remember being told that they had taken 'the pledge' but only knew that that meant that they did not smoke and drink and that later in our childhoods we thought it funny that they drank

Crabbie's Green Ginger wine at Christmas, thinking it was a cordial and not alcoholic.

I would be frightened to get too much into religion or our history, but thinking of how powerfully my dad hated the Sunday services, his almost rejection of his faith, and later on my fervent evangelism, replaced by fervent atheism, now superseded by my conviction that I am evil and a devil. I wonder, but only idly, if there are causes and effects for such lineage that I am not really aware of and if I follow a line influenced by my forebears.

My dad's parents moved to Devon after the war. From what I can gather, it was a good move. He had found, to his and his family's surprise, that he was very clever. He flourished in school and spent what seemed to be an idyllic time roaming the countryside with friends. As he grew up, the railway sets and bicycles of childhood, some of which were passed on to me as a child, with no idea of their history and which disappeared with all my other possessions when my marriage failed, were replaced by a yearning for motorbikes and cars and flying.

I still haven't ridden a motorbike! My dad was driving his motorbike to school at sixteen and parking it so that it would not be seen when he walked into class. He worked in the summer holidays as a beach photographer, taking the pictures, developing and enlarging them in a studio he made in his attic.

At the same time he joined the Air Training Corps and applied for a flying scholarship. He says he was hooked when he started flying Gypsy Moths and that he received his pilot's licence when he was seventeen, before he got his driving licence.

My mum, I remember even less of. She talked of swimming in the sea in every sort of weather and how exciting it was to get caught in the undertow of wild waves. She talked of an old navy torpedo boat that she and her fellow Sea Scouts used to do whatever Sea Scouts do in such places and she talked of wonderful jam sandwiches on that boat and of the navy recruits she mixed with and of becoming a nurse like her sister did too and also of some of the huge mistakes her mum made with their money. I think her mum wanted her and her sister to work in a nursing home she planned to set up, but that they wouldn't. I know that finally, her mum spent most of the working life she had, when I knew her, as some sort of lady's companion with various people and that her husband, Fred, acted as an engineer, cleaning massive boilers of asbestos and also living in rented rooms.

My dad went to university to study petroleum engineering. His life and what he did is such a contrast to mine – do have a look at these small extracts from his memoir:

The third and last place I went to was Jabel Fahood... in the Trucial, Oman, as another part of my introduction to the reality of the oil business. This was an exploration base, miles out in the desert, with trucks for seismic survey and a mobile rig to drill test holes. Just after I arrived there one of the teams came back with bullet holes in the trucks, they were so far off the beaten track that the local Bedouin had not even seen vehicles... An early lesson there was ALWAYS to check your shoes for scorpions before putting them on – on a couple of occasions I was glad that I did.

... As the new man there I was introduced to the local Sheik, straight out of Lawrence of Arabia; aquiline, black tent with a rifle slung along the roof ridge and beautiful carpets over the sand. One of the most impressive people I have ever met. His palace was in an oasis a couple of hundred miles away, I asked him why he was living on the site rather than in his home. He said simply: 'My people are here, where else should I be?' Mind you, he was driven back every month to his palace for a few days.

The next year he went to Canada:

Towards the end of my stay in Canada I had enough cash to stay for 3 days in Jasper Park Lodge, an outstanding resort hotel, the smartest

*log cabins you could imagine with every amenity you could think of –
they claimed that at any time they could assemble enough guests for a
quorum of the United States or Canadian Senate. I stayed in one of the
golfer's log cabins, not exactly roughing it but not the same standard
of luxury as the main cabins, hardly a problem since you just walked
a hundred yards or so to the lounges or restaurants which were very
upmarket. At lunchtime on the first day I was grabbed by one of the
golfers, who was panic struck about the snoring coming from his room.
It was very loud snoring and came from a black bear that had snuggled
down on his bed. He looked very comfortable; the staff finally convinced
the bear to move out.*

When I read my dad's account of his childhood and his early years,
I do not know what to think. He says elsewhere that he felt his parents
were selfish and that he inherited that trait from them but I don't know,
maybe we are all selfish in different ways.

I see someone who had a joy for life, who was busy learning, meeting
new and wonderful people and situations. I was going to say someone
full of confidence, and he does appear to be that in his memoir, but I
remember one day, many years ago, when I was in my late adolescence,
one of those rare times that he gave me advice that I listened to, even if I
ignored it. He told me that he had always been shy, that he had struggled
to speak to people and to socialise but that he forced himself to do it and
never looked back afterwards.

The more I think about how he was at that age, I see a person I would
have craved to have been and also loathed with all my heart. At that age
I was just learning that I didn't want to live; I was deliberately failing at
university and as far as I could tell, this was to stop the embarrassment of
failing because I couldn't do the work; far from gaining the confidence
to charm and entertain and find new adventures, I was withdrawing and
I still remain silent in company.

But then, it was just after university that I made my first friends;

found my first glimpse of the need to make a difference. I had no money and was busy rejecting my middle class inheritance. I was living in a single room, came late to girlfriends, came very late to conversation or parties; my parties usually involved me calling an ambulance for my friend, Vaughn, who had learning disabilities and once he had drunk too much would have grand mal fits or take overdoses of pills or both. The number of dark streets and closed pubs with Vaughn jerking on the ground, pissing his pants. It doesn't really compare to my dad dining on the Isle de France when crossing the Atlantic.

But we were both growing in our own similar ways. In those days I was rejecting my background and all it stood for, just as my dad was leaving behind his upbringing and reaching for something that seemed better and for him, more exciting.

I wonder why I compare myself so much to my dad and not to my mum? It is she who taught me the biggest lessons in life: about compassion and humour and most especially about the optimism of celebrating what we have. She has shown me so much about how to put up with the worst that life can throw at you and to keep functioning. If I had wanted to emulate someone it should have been her and yet my dad was always the centre of everything. We, his wife and children, circled round him like satellites. I think maybe very, very late in life I am realising the effect of patriarchy on all of us; that I compare myself and my achievements to him, when I could have learnt so much more about relationships and the things that are truly valuable from my mum.

Wendy has recently taken over that task too, but it takes so long to understand and come to terms with. I am still puffed with pride when I am asked to do a piece of work that is prestigious or to write something people will read with interest. And although Wendy says it is family and friends and how we treated each other and what we did together that I will remember when I am old and dying, rather than what article was published or mountain I climbed, I still look back on those markers of success with glimmers of regret at what I haven't done, and with pomposity at what I can list to show the success I could almost be said to have had, despite this schizophrenia stuff.

2020—FEBRUARY—ME AND MY MENTAL HEALTH—SHORT BREAK AT KNOCKDERRY CASTLE

We are used to it now, we have had practice; even gained some patience with the system. After ten years you would hope we would have.

Each tribunal is different; contains its own surprises, its own memorable events but, to be honest, in a way I find painful. That last one, a scant two months ago, I can hardly remember it.

You would think that going to what is, in effect, a court, would stick in your memory, but try as I might, I can't remember the detail at all. Of course, I remember the decision but then Wendy had told me beforehand that it was inevitable and I both did and did not believe her, was both reassured and dismayed.

I remember that we went to the wrong building to start with and that this time, unlike last time, we did not have to hang around trying to get attention, did not have to have the security guards in the room explained to us. The person who greeted us was nice; she seemed a kind person but slightly sad. The room she got us to wait in was so much better than that last cramped, untidy room of two years ago.

Because we were first, we got the comfy chairs. It seemed wrong when the psychiatrist and social worker came in and had to sit in the plastic chairs. I almost got up and asked them to take my one and then thought, *No, not today.*

It is strange to sit waiting, opposing parties as it were. Sitting together, awkwardly, in the same room before being summoned to the panel in the next room; exchanging pleasantries.

Wendy is very good at this; she draws people out, connects with them, tries to make them feel at ease.

There is a familiarity to this that I am both weary of and delighted to encounter. I know these people, have known them for a number of years. Though I know little of who they are, what they like, what their families are like, what they wish for and what they fear, at least I know their mannerisms and am beginning to sense something of them as people and not just as combatants. They are no longer impersonal officials mapping out my destiny.

To be clear, though, at these moments I do see them as my enemies. I will hate it when they talk about my private life and my past and my inner thoughts and desires in front of strangers who will decide on my future. Although I will try to smile and laugh, my leg will be jiggering up and down and I will be staring out the window as people speak about me; doing my very best to look at the sky, the trees, the seagulls and crows. Wanting not to be here, not hearing all these words. Being there but doing my very, very best to not be there; even though I came willingly, hoping to bear witness to what was being done to me. At times I will want to cry and at times I will want to hug my love and at times I will hear my psychiatrist saying things about my past that are just plain incorrect and I will think: *I could challenge this, make them seem foolish and ill prepared* and yet I do not.

I maintain my silence and let my leg jigger away again as it does at such times, while I stare out at that dark silhouette of the tree outside the window. I look at the low building opposite, the parked cars; staff and patients ambling around while we remain inside for this little, very personal, mini drama.

I have given them a prepared statement in which I accept there are different ways of seeing the world and in which I acknowledge that I do not know what decision I want them to reach.

Because life is complicated, justice and rights are complicated. If I have my way, and I am far from sure I want my way, I will be free to stop my treatment and if I do, going by the evidence of past years, my life will be at risk. The darkness and the terror and the thoughts that I now only have at two in the morning will be there all the time, and instead of worrying about the effect on the driver of the train if I step on the tracks at Queen Street, I will instead see the rush of air that heralds all that fast, so solid, so final metal as my salvation, my oblivion, my release from what I subject those I love to, by existing. Or else I will be back to the filled petrol cans, the razor blades, the pills and the electricity; the scalding water.

And if I don't have my way, I will have to open my shirt every two weeks for that jag and the drugs that, as far as I am concerned, stop me being real; stop me really, really knowing how much I am harming the world and those I love. I will continue with this claggy twilight, where I struggle to think, to brighten and laugh, where I am *still* but in all the worst ways. I will open my shirt and, since that time a few months ago, worry that with the clogging of the scar tissue from the years of injections, they will again have to use two hands on the syringe, such is the resistance in my shoulder to the liquid. Or that they will even have to give up, remove the needle, stuck so deep in my muscle, and ask me to lower my trousers instead, for access to a site where it is so much easier to drug me.

I remember I liked the psychiatrist on the panel. She seemed interested, but Wendy didn't like her, thought she took us on tangents. I think the legal person and the lay person were nice but I really don't know. I cannot see or hear them in my memory any more. I liked the humanity and regret of my social worker and could see that my doctor was trying his best, but we knew what would happen.

After ten years of this, it is easy to predict the result. Although each time I think they will at last realise that I am not ill, not what they say I am, and each time Wendy laughs at my naivety. We also laugh when she says that she agrees with them too.

Twenty five years of schizophrenia and thirty five years of admissions to hospitals... When, with each admission, you are followed everywhere

51

you go; where the light is not turned out for weeks at a time so that you yearn for darkness, to sleep without being stared at. Where the door from the ward is barred to you; the feel of grass, the fresh air of the hills and the lochside become a distant memory. Where you have to learn the complex dance of going to the toilet or having a shower while the nurses watch; trying to work out which ones are the least awkward to be naked in front of.

I can begin to understand why some in the United Nations say that this is cruel and degrading treatment and akin to torture. I can both see and not see this.

Because without this cruel and degrading treatment; without my restriction, now provided in the community, I wouldn't get to kiss Wendy every morning. I wouldn't cuddle her daughter after school and giggle when her son says something so dry and cutting it becomes hilarious. I wouldn't walk the dog by the shore, listening to the lap of the waves, taking photos of the sunken sugar boat in the Firth and the hills deeper into Argyll. I wouldn't feel the wind and the sun, the cool smirr of rain; smell the sea air; hear the bird song, the geese, the swans and oystercatchers. Witness my Wendy's wonderful, optimistic humor as we peer around us at the cumbersome herons; the bobbing seals.

I wouldn't be here, and if I was, by some faint chance, my life would not be the joy it is just now. I would not work or write. I would not cook or listen to the radio in the early morning. I would not laugh or sit at the table outside, with my whisky, in the summer. I would not wake in the snoring room with Dash the dog cuddled up to me in the morning. I would not annoy the family by asking them again and again what they want me to cook them for breakfast and lunch and tea. I would not. I just would not.

Because we are used to this and although we have developed a patience with it, we know, when the verdict is handed down, we will still be halted and dulled and shocked; despite knowing this will happen and has done so for year after year after year.

This will happen as long as I say into the silence, "I want to die." As long as I deny I have schizophrenia, as long as I refuse my drugs.

And because, when we walk out of the room after their verdict, I will be shaky and wanting to escape, Wendy has booked us a night in a hotel on a strange peninsular of bizarre and wonderful houses; a place of peace and calm and distraction and rare luxury.

And delightfully, when we arrive, we find that she has made a mistake and has actually booked us into the Airbnb in the castle perched on the cliff above the hotel.

It is wonderful, and so incongruous that I forget the tribunal, the medical reports, all those ponderous serious expressions. That burden of words, evidence, that burden of decision-making where my existence is being decided on.

We have three rooms. A wonderful bed, views over the loch, sofas, a fridge and television, a dining table, a washing machine and Dash the dog galumphing all over the place; us frightened he will get his muddy paws on the bed.

I have my whisky; Wendy has her diet coke and tea. We pause, sleep before dinner, cuddled together. When I take Dash out for his wee in the evening, the sight of a flock of deer grazing in the castle grounds delights me, sparks him. They run away into the dark; he goes frantic.

Later we go down the dark, muddy, leafy track, using our phones as torches, to the hotel we thought we had been booked into originally.

We eat in the room reserved for dog owners; talk with fellow diners about their day. Try to be polite when someone says how great Brexit is and how bad independence would be.

We delight in the treat of food and wine and leave the 'section', that tribunal that goes on and on, far, far behind. So far behind I don't even think about what our dining companions would think if they knew what happened to us today, if they knew why we were here. So far, that I forget that I am on the committee that is reviewing the very legislation I have just been sectioned under, yet again.

In the morning, the sun shines. There is snow on the hills of the Cowal peninsula opposite us.

Wendy is still kissing me; Dash can still smell the deer; the young children of the castle owner are bashful when they see us outside. There are snowdrops. There will be more mornings like this.

And are we being patient with them? Those that decide on my future, my life? Or them with us?

2019—FEBRUARY—SANDY—LAST DAYS

It was after Christmas that Sandy's new-found energy after he stopped his chemotherapy dwindled away. Initially we were still coming round every evening to make tea for him, to watch telly and tell stories about work and about Dash the dog. The children still played computer games, watched *Scooby Doo*, ate biscuits and drew pictures. Dash still emptied the bins and had to be chased for the tissues and chocolate wrappers.

But Sandy wanted less and less to eat, his car had been sitting unused in front of the house for months – a constant reminder of what was going to happen. We were exhausted, I remember that. The months and months of false happiness after his operation, well, not false, we were happy, but it was like a false war, where you laugh and dance knowing the invasion is imminent. The daily visits to make tea and provide some humour, that brief spell when we took to taking him to Barca's when he seemed, by the greatest of illogicalities, to be getting better. That stopped.

Sandy – I can't remember what prompted him to ask it, it would have been what we all knew really but did not quite want to – asked his nurse how long he had left to live and she told him no more than two weeks.

He didn't expect that, was shocked. So was Wendy. She said, how could we make him laugh and chatter with us when we all had this final news?

Wendy took time off work, so did Peter. Sandy had been referred to the end of life team but they did not seem to be arriving at all. We wondered where they had got to, wondered if we would have to deal with all this on our own.

The children began to hate coming round, they hated opening the door to his house, worried each time that he might have died. Sandy was now upstairs all the time.

We had someone up there most of the time. Sometimes Charlotte would come upstairs, sometimes she would cry. James refused to come up at all. I think he still said he thought his papa would get better but he became very quiet. They hated us when we picked them up from school and said we were off to see Sandy. We had to bribe them with trips to McDonald's and with pizza for tea when, as usual, we were late home, with the dog needing walked and the children needing to do their homework.

We were giving him whatever he felt he could drink or eat, mainly Barrs cream soda with lots of ice in and sometimes ice cream.

Wendy still managed to get him to laugh. While Sandy so often said, "It is what it is," and I nodded solemnly and sadly, Wendy could witter away and bring laughter into his life. That seemed so special and was also such a big thing for her to find the courage and energy to do.

I remember one evening we needed some help for him and phoned round and round, being referred backwards and forwards and ultimately never getting the help we needed.

Going for a pee became difficult and needed planning, Sandy would prepare well in advance, rocking himself into position so that he could get his legs out of the bed, get into a sitting position and then, leaning on

Peter or me, walk very, very slowly to the toilet where we would help him take his trousers down to wee.

We had begun to stay overnight in the house, staying there twenty four hours a day. Peter had taken the futon in the spare room downstairs and either he or I would sleep on it, going up for brief natters, to help Sandy have a drink or to give him his medication and wait for him to sleep again.

Sandy had been changing his stoma bag, but now it was becoming too much for him. He taught me how to do it, but I only actually had to do it once before he finally agreed to the home carers coming in.

That one time I did it, I remember I was very nervous. He took me through the whole routine, time and time again, until I knew exactly what I was meant to do. It wasn't that hard but maybe not the ideal job for squeamish people. I remember the night after that, putting up a post on Twitter asking why family were having to change stoma bags.

Finally, the end of life team arrived, as did the home carers, and they were somehow superb. Sandy had stopped shaving, did not want to change his bedclothes or his sheets but within an hour he was shaved, washed, clean, saying he felt so much better.

He was very ambivalent about having them there; said we could manage fine, but we were less sure. He was also ambivalent about what he wanted to happen, hospital? Hospice? Death at home? In the end he opted for hospice; they said he was unlikely to get into it but would refer him anyway.

Sandy had made it clear that he wanted nothing much at all for his funeral: no service, no flowers, no announcements. Nothing.

Some people might think this was unconventional and brutal, but I think it suited Wendy, and Peter too. They didn't want a service, with people to entertain, food to give out, condolences to be given and accepted. It seemed unnecessary and false to them.

He also wanted us to sell off his huge book collection and give the proceeds to the children.

For some reason, he thought I had done far more to help than I needed to and asked Wendy and Peter to make sure that after he died I should be given whisky for a year. It pleased me. It also pleased me that Wendy kept on saying she didn't know how she would have managed without my help.

It will sound wrong, considering this was someone's death that we were dealing with, but my biggest fear all along was that I would not be able to support Wendy and the children enough. That with the death of her dad would come the death of our relationship and yet somehow, despite my failing words and inability to provide humour, I did what she needed most of the time. I was so incredibly relieved at that.

One Friday I was at the house alone, while Wendy was looking after the children at home. Peter was at home asleep, after being at the house the night before, and Sharon (his partner) was at work.

All was sort of as it had been for the last few days, but in the late afternoon we had the most innocuous crisis. Sandy needed to go to the toilet and was just too weak to get out of bed. We had a bizarre and slightly humorous conversation. First of all we tried to decide if I could carry him there and decided that would be too risky, in case I dropped him, and then we practiced piling up his store of nappies around him which he had been using for some time to deal with the discharge after his bowel operation, but that seemed very unsatisfactory too.

Finally, we decided that I should chop up a fizzy juice bottle as an improvised potty. We both laughed at my effort, although Sandy was in pain and tired. The improvised potty didn't work either.

The second call I made on Sandy's behalf over these weeks was to try to get help to let Sandy have the wee he desperately wanted to have. I couldn't get through to the end of life care team and when I did, they were out elsewhere. When I got through to the health visitors they were flummoxed and did not know what to suggest. Finally, I spoke to a doctor who said he would come out.

And he did, and pretty quickly at that. He had a long chat with Sandy, told him the options were to be carried to the toilet by us two or, much easier, just peeing the bed. With that, he suggested to Sandy that now was the time to go into hospital and Sandy chose to wee the bed.

We hadn't known how Sandy would deal with this time when it came, but somehow the doctor almost seemed to give him permission to accept this; permission to sort of stop.

I was quite shocked when the doctor phoned the hospital. They were extremely reluctant to let Sandy come in and kept on saying couldn't we, as family, look after him, and the doctor kept on saying we were beyond the stage of managing at home and in the end nearly had to insist on an admission. Had to become very assertive indeed.

He left about five pm, saying that the ambulance might take a couple of hours as they were really stretched at the moment but that it should be there by seven.

Sandy wanted to be left alone and went back to sleep while I waited for the ambulance. Peter was due to take over from me later in the evening but the ambulance still hadn't arrived by nine pm, when he arrived. The next day he told us that it finally arrived at three in the morning.

It seemed to me that this was an undignified last few hours at his house and, although the controller person checked in occasionally and apologised, it would have been good if Sandy had been picked up at a reasonable time and given the chance to sleep in some comfort instead of in a urine-soaked bed.

Peter disappeared home to sleep and I went into the hospital in the morning to see how Sandy was. I took in a few of the things we thought he might want. It seems silly now. The pyjamas, dressing gown, the Irn Bru and so on. None of it was touched.

The ward was a bit shocking, the people in it looking so ill. I remember one man: emaciated, his head flung right back, his mouth wide open, breathing noisily and with difficulty.

Sandy was hardly awake and said he just wanted to sleep so I stayed just moments and went back home to Wendy.

Around three that afternoon we got a call from the hospital saying it would be a good idea to come in as Sandy had taken a turn for the worse. To our relief, Tom, (the children's dad) had just got home and was able to pick up the children and Dash.

I remember so vividly that walk up to the hospital in the Vale. We were walking up the hill from the lower car park and Wendy broke down as we turned the corner to the building and the ward he was in, not sure if she could face going up to the ward or how she would cope with seeing her dad. She cuddled up to me and then found something in her that allowed her to take her next steps; found a very shaky laugh.

On the ward, Sandy was only just conscious as we sat with him. I remember small bits of humour and tenderness: how he almost burst out laughing when I was wittering about the difficulties of using lettuce in stir fries and how, when the nurse asked if he would like tea with sweeteners, he said enthusiastically and loudly that that would be a great idea when, as far as we knew, he nearly never had tea and certainly not with sweeteners.

They gave him ice cream that one of us fed him and that he enjoyed, and then we talked; sat, talked to each other and Sandy, looked at the other visitors and patients.

Wendy had been trying to phone Peter but he was not answering his phone, presumably still asleep from the night before. Eventually she called Sharon who got through to him.

He arrived around seven and Sharon, later, sometime between eight and nine. Sharon had texted to ask if we wanted anything and we had said we wanted nothing but found we were delighted when she arrived with sandwiches and juice and cakes and crisps.

By this time we had all been moved off the ward and into a separate room. Sandy was peaceful, sleeping mostly, and we were all gathered around the bed. The room was a terrible mess of glaring lights to start with, but then they switched off all the lights, leaving just a faint one by the bed, making the room feel warm and soft and homely.

If I were a person with a good memory and with more skill than I have, this book would just be about those last hours of Sandy's life.

It was the most intense, focused time I have ever spent. In some ways, the most peaceful and the most beautiful of my life and in others, just horrendous.

We did not know we were going to do it, or even that we were doing it, but we were holding a vigil and we were trying to hold Sandy with love and warmth.

We talked through the night, just softly. We told jokes, talked about memories of our different childhoods and adulthoods, calling the nurse when Sandy seemed to need more medication. Talking to Sandy, watching him, loving him. Munching on our Hula Hoops and flapjacks. I remember I reverted to childhood and ate my Hula Hoops off the tips of my fingers. I remember how we began to wish Sharon had brought more food in when our snacks ran out and how she had known to take the snacks in because, not long before, she had been through the same thing with her gran, who had brought her and her twin sister up.

We talked about Peter's guinea pigs and how he would be better getting a dog. We talked of Lewis (Sharon's young son) and how he was managing in school and recovering from the operation that had gone wrong. The times when Wendy referred to herself as Super Wendy and the squabbles she had with Peter during their childhood. We talked about Sharon's gran. We went to Disneyland again with the children. We revisited the time Peter went motorboating, drunk, in the middle of the night on Loch Lomond. The time I nearly got run down by a ship in the mid Atlantic. We talked of the pain of me not seeing my son, Calum, and the pain of Peter not seeing his daughter, Abi, and how sad it was that Sandy hadn't been able to see her for months and months. And how disastrous separations can be, how bitter some people can be. We glowed about how well Wendy and Tom had managed their separation. We giggled about the time when Peter was young, on holiday with the family at a caravan park, and how he went into the wrong caravan. Giggled again about when Peter got Wendy to drink a glass of orange juice in one go, having neglected to tell her it was laced with tabasco sauce. We giggled, in a slightly shocked way, at Wendy's escapades as a child; we talked about work and the politics of work. At one point we were talking about visiting Pompeii and at another, about how Peter disciplines Lewis and how Sophie (Sharon's daughter) is doing; about Sharon's sister, Clare, and her family.

This long, long, rambling conversation, punctuated with jokes and laughter and queries about how long we could make the Hula Hoops last, and all the time we were speaking, we were watching Sandy; the soft conversation, the warmth of quiet laughter and the room, it made everything feel calm and peaceful.

At one point Sharon went out to persuade the nurse that Sandy needed medication again but it took some time to get permission from the duty doctor and shortly after, Wendy and I were quite shocked to hear there was only one doctor on duty for the whole hospital. Anyway, they put him on a morphine pump, sending us out while they did it.

Because Peter and Sharon worked in the hospital, in the labs, we went down to the small kitchen they used and drank coffee, and severely startled one of their colleagues who walked in, expecting to see no one there, and who initially just saw me, a stranger, drinking coffee in the middle of the night in her kitchen, through the window on the door.

Around eleven, I left the ward and sat out in a shrub-lined courtyard, surrounded by trees, needing some space and fresh air. I sat in the dark night, listening to the birds and the wind, getting some cool air, some relief. People would pass, talking. The leaves in the tree rustled and oh! the coolness, the freshness and the darkness after the hospital. That was so good.

Another time, later that night, I wanted to go out again but the doors were locked by then. I wandered up and down the stairs, looking at the various health posters, trying to find space, a place to calm my mind but couldn't find it.

Later still, Wendy went to the toilet and we were sent out of the room when they needed to do something to Sandy. She came out, saw us walking down the corridor and assumed Sandy had just died. She crumpled when she saw us, got hugged and was then filled with laughter as we talked about how we could have kidded her that her dad had actually died. It seemed funny at the time, I really don't know why it seemed funny now, but at the time it did; it made us laugh and laugh, maybe slightly hysterically.

Around one in the morning, when the doors to the outside had long since been locked, we kept on hearing the most beautiful birdsong. It was wonderful, so beautiful; such a lovely, lovely sound to hear while we sat in that quiet room. We kept wondering what bird would be singing away in the middle of the night, were completely baffled. Why on earth would a songbird be singing when the rest of the world was asleep?

Then there was the nurse, sometimes coming in to give us a cup of tea or to check Sandy's pain relief.

In the twilight of the room, all there was, was the hushed conversation between us, the stories, the jokes, the laughter, the confessions. And always, someone checking that Sandy was ok, checking whether he was in pain, if he needed something. Even though he was mainly unconscious we were somehow pretty sure that we did know how he was, could pick up when he was peaceful and when he was slightly more uncomfortable; a tiny bit more agitated.

Outside our room it was all bright lights, noise and whiteness, but here, we were in a pool of peace with birdsong accompanying us.

Sandy's breathing became shallower and shallower throughout the night and his times approaching consciousness less and less, and I don't know if we were tired, it was like some other place, another dimension where the thought of sleep hardly occurred to us.

Not long before he died, he raised his arms slowly above his head and then relaxed them, having hardly moved for hours; he seemed to be looking at something wonderful and then in the final minutes, he breathed so softly.

We were talking quietly but all of us were watching him, and then we stopped talking. I think we all knew the moment he went. When those, tiny, faint breaths just stopped and we paused, watched, and almost held our own breath, stilled our own muscles.

Sharon broke the silence and said, "I think he's gone."

And we agreed.

Someone went to get the nurse and we were ushered into another room with some redundant machinery in it. They gave us tea and told us to stay there while they did whatever needed done to Sandy.

I think we were exhausted and I don't know if anyone cried or hugged or anything. I just remember the long, narrow room, the mismatched chairs and the bits of hospital equipment.

The nurse, who we had built into our heads as a Nurse Ratched character, and made jokes about throughout the night, had actually been very sensitive in a brusque way. I think there was something lovely when she said something like, "The poor wee darling."

Something loving, although she must have witnessed death almost every day.

She told us we could go and view his body, pay our respects, but no one apart from me wanted to go and see him. They said that that wasn't Sandy and was not how they wanted to remember him.

I remember standing in the room. He was so still and so small and his skin seemed to have shrunk around his temples into big indents. I didn't say much, just, "Goodbye Sandy. You were a lovely man, a lovely man." I felt tears prickling my eyes, wiped them away and went back to the others.

It was five in the morning. We drove back home with the dawn approaching. Up over the hill that we had been back and forth over every day, for the last six months or more, to see Sandy at his house.

We saw the lights of Greenock and Gourock, where my friend Jen's parents live, and the lights near Dunoon, near where my sister would have been sleeping. Saw the patterns of light on the dark of the Clyde, crossed the bumpy cattle grid, went down the winding road in the woods besides St Peter's Seminary and into Cardross and home.

I can't remember some of the basic things. Did Wendy want me to sleep beside her as she sometimes does when she is upset, or were we so tired that we collapsed into our separate beds?

Did we sit up for a time? Did Wendy have a cup of tea or me a whisky? I don't know. Just that we were stunned and exhausted, that somehow we had witnessed something very beautiful and very, very sad at the same time.

I don't know when we woke up the next day, but I do remember walking the dog at some point. Tom must have looked after him that night, and suddenly I remembered what the birdsong had been; that of a blackbird, of course:

'Blackbird singing in the dead of night!'

I googled the lyrics and found out the song was meant to be about civil rights, but those lyrics also make me think of death and release too; seemed somehow appropriate.

And that was the end, in a way. Sandy did not believe in God at all, saw death very much as a return to nothingness. But I wonder if it was also a beginning, even if it was only that release from fear and pain, that long, everlasting, soft, smooth sleep. I hope so.

I was privileged to know Sandy, to be allowed to be a part of his family for those last few years, privileged to have been allowed to help in some way.

I can't quite remember what happened next. Wendy would have told Tom. Did she tell the children? Or did Tom? I think she did.

Tom kept them with him for the weekend, I think. Charlotte was brave enough to go to Orlaith's birthday party the following day, managed to find some pleasure in that.

We met Peter and Sharon later that day for lunch at the Queen of the Loch. I think it all felt a bit unreal but there was this strong feeling amongst all of us that those last few hours were as good a way of dying as you could possibly have and also a sense of connection between us all.

March

2021—MARCH—WENDY—ORDERING THE WILDNESS OF THE DAY

They do dance, those windsurfers, don't they? That sea is silver; the bay has lines of tiny whitecaps stretched across it in ragged rows and the two windsurfers, with their bright red translucent sails, are bouncing across the waves, the masts bobbing this way and that in the wind; spray flying in their wake.

I am just doing my normal dog walk. I was down by the sea earlier, where, in the lea of the isthmus, the sea is still and soft and laps just gently on the turf of the land because the tide is so high. There are veils of rain on the far hills, there is still that roar from the trees on the windward side that you get on a windy day, but there is also sunshine and brightness.

Not so long ago I would have been thinking of crossing continents to see you, but now you are always here. You came up to my room this morning, just as Desert Island Discs was finishing. You bounced into bed, were delighted that Dash the dog got so excited to see you, bounding onto the bed, tail wagging, licking your face, his big paws carelessly placed on my cheek and my chest. You rolled him on his back and cuddled him tightly and then you cuddled me and asked if it was time to get up.

There is something endearing about these times; you come all the way upstairs for a two minute cuddle which I am sure you want, but really, you just love it when you can sit on the sofa while I make breakfast for you. I love it too; to be needed sometimes, to make the morning start well; what better feeling could there be?

I think a curlew just flew over, all skinny wings and a tumbling flight, as though it was being half bowled over by the wind and half doing aerobatics. I know the name of very few things really. Sometimes I cling to the idea of learning so that I could know why that bird makes that noise or the why the wee lambs are so still in the field beside their mothers, or why the flock of geese chose that field near the railway to stop in or why it is you love me, or just what love really is.

Navigating life and making sense of it. I have an inkling that that could be good; to shape it to my design and pleasure. To carve a route between the bewildering trees and mountains, to know what is lovable and what is not only irritating but quite off-putting. To understand why wee Charlotte says every day that she loves me and gangs up on Wendy when she is teasing me, and to realise why James sometimes does the opposite but tells his mum that he likes me but that I make him shy.

I do not understand such things. The world and my place in it remain a mystery to me. Why that bird tumbled in the wind above my head, I have no idea. Why you like to snuggle up to me in the evening and why you find me funny despite myself, I haven't a clue.

But, shortly, I will get back into the car and drive to Craigendoran to pick you up from Paula's garden, where you will smile at me and offer me a sticky bun and agree with Paula when she says I did the right thing in calling the ambulance when we did not know if you were having a panic attack or if your UTI had flared out of control and I will feel like I belong here. That even though I do not understand it, I fit in; that I am a part of the family. I am Dash the dog's daddy; Mummy's boyfriend who the children can't remember not being there. The one who puts the bins out and gets excited each time they are all due to go out on the same day, much to the amusement of my loving, uncomprehending family.

But first let us linger to watch the windsurfers; the spray, the wild bright sky, their adrenaline-fuelled adventure. I am on a similar adventure, not adrenaline-fuelled, but yesterday, when I came downstairs and found Charlotte curled under the downie, Wendy putting the pillow over her ears as I made the children's lunch and her coffee, how drowsily she drank it while tussle-haired, more asleep than awake, Charlotte nuzzled into her for a few extra minutes before it was time to get ready for school. That everyday occurrence is the greatest adventure. I still don't realise that it is real and will continue for day after day, just as my walks by the sea with Dash the dog will, and that every morning the rooks will wake me as they too prepare for the day.

I do not need to learn any more: the tumbling bird was a tumbling bird. Wendy's kiss and Wendy's smile were just that: a kiss and a smile.

2021—MARCH—MY JOURNAL

This March is typical of any year. There are days where the air is balmy and we find no need to wear coats, moments when I think I might be able to put the washing out on the line and then come gales and driving rain and snow on the hills.

I love this time of year as the snowdrops come out and the daffodils blossom. And in some ways so much has already happened this year.

I had a jag where the drug wouldn't go in again and the nurse had to go out to get help to find out what to do. I can't quite remember what it was that she ended up doing, but it was all solved. It meant I forgot to ask her about the psychological therapy they keep on half promising.

Mum got vaccinated ages ago, although she is still due her second jag, and so did Wendy's mum. I am one of the lower priorities but because there is a very high mortality rate for people with schizophrenia with the virus, I was a bit of a priority and suddenly found myself getting my jag in early March. It was so well organised. A phone call. Lining up in a fast-moving queue at the sports hall, being asked a few questions, getting given a leaflet, walking up for the jag I didn't even feel, sitting down for five minutes and then going home.

Initially, I didn't think I was affected at all by the vaccine, but by the time morning came I was fuzzy in my body. This is a lovely side effect,

I thought. Not much later, I wondered if I had a very bad hangover, not long after that, as the aches and the headache and the chills mounted, I wondered if I had caught Covid at the same time as getting the vaccine. Not long after that I was back in bed! I had a miserable day, but later in the evening, suddenly, it all subsided and life began to feel good again and Wendy commented that I must have been very busy building up antibodies!

I still dream about my dad. Last night, I found myself stumbling onto a memorial ground somehow looking over towards Vietnam to commemorate victims of the war. There were American soldiers all over the place, looking sad and solemn and pretty fed up that I had walked all over a specially raked-over patch of sand. My dad was beside me and he sat down beside the soldiers and said his name and rank in the Air Force and saluted them, which pleased them. They got talking about the guns he would have had in his helicopter (he never flew helicopters), they had slang words for them but he only knew them by their proper names and this made them smile.

I do look forward to these dreams. In some ways I think I am getting to know him better in my sleep. I am not really. I am making up an image of him in my mind and I do not know if it bears any relation to reality, but in it he is much more vulnerable, much more open and mild mannered. I like the person I meet here very much and think he may have been someone I could have had as a very, very good friend, rather than as a dad with the different relationships that implies.

I remember those years of my later adolescence and the debates we had that I hated, and wish that I had been stronger, could have seen them as testing and exciting, rather than as an attack on my very fragile sense of self.

This time, three years ago, I was down visiting my dad and my mum. I was being spoilt with the bedroom upstairs which looks out onto the lawn and the cherry tree.

In those days my dad was really beginning to struggle more and more and needed more and more help from my mum with dressing and basic hygiene. I want the fact that you can still love and still live well when life is precarious to be reflected in the reality that it is also a difficult, grimy, unappealing existence and that we are not always as kind or as loving as we would wish to be. My dad could get fed up with the care my mum tirelessly gave him and my mum could get fed up that he did not know how to express his gratitude and love when sometimes she very much needed it. I want these small indignities celebrated in a weird way, glimpses of Mum dressing Dad were incredibly tender to me, despite the very indignities I mentioned that were central at the same time.

I feel disconnected from these times somehow, they already seem a long time ago. Maybe, because of Covid and lockdown, it seems like I am talking about another age rather than just a few years ago. Because of course, this time, only a year ago, lockdown started and we learnt a whole new set of rules. So recent! I remember all those news programs. I think the children thought we had entered the end days of the world and that we would all die very soon indeed.

Charlotte had finally managed time in her own bed, some months after her papa's death, but with Covid she returned to her mum's bed. James would get frightened and go up to the top floor where they slept, later on at night. I started phoning my mum every night and wondered why I had not done so while Dad was alive.

I have a feeling that it was also about this time, in 2018, that I finally got officially divorced from my wife. She made it difficult to the end, refusing to accept and sign for the divorce papers until we had to pay a few hundred pounds to do something that meant the papers had been served on her. Considering that she got a settlement of at least one hundred thousand pounds more than I think she should have, you would have thought she would have been quick to sign, but then maybe she knew just how much I would have dreaded the battle of trying to get anything approaching a fifty-fifty divorce.

To grumble about that! More important was Sandy at the same time in 2018: walking into a friend's shop, not being recognised and then, after the enthusiastic greeting, having to explain the cancer, introduce me for the first time and at the same time say he probably wouldn't see his friend again. How did Sandy do such things in a few short, gentle sentences? Such things amaze me and teach me the lesson that bitterness is useless.

2020—MARCH—MENTAL HEALTH AND ME— REALITY CHECK

I want to talk about the assumptions I used to make with my companions and comrades about our lives and how we interpreted them.

Was it really thirty years ago that we made our own 'Glad to be Mad' t-shirts? And did I really wear one? Self conscious and yet outrageously pleased with myself!

Was it twenty years ago that I was talking joyfully about 'Mad Pride' to a friend who said, "Why would you be proud of madness? I am proud of friends with a mental illness, but proud of illness?"

I paused, because sometimes I do listen. I remembered those times of absolute agony; a hell of feeling and not feeling I had never felt before; I wondered if she was right.

I remember, how long ago? Maybe fifteen years? Another friend described how she saw her experience of psychosis as a spiritual awakening; a blossoming into a new state of awareness. Those wonderful insights into her life; how she looked forward to the morning when she drew the curtains so that she could have that half hour conversation with her voices before going into work.

I thrilled at that, but in the back of my mind I remembered. Those weeks of unutterable struggle and paranoia that have besieged her for years. I still think of her warmth and her belief in something grander than the mundanity of illness with pleasure, but would I want a spiritual awakening like hers?

I don't know. I spend most of my time trying not to believe those thoughts that besiege me; my certainty that I am a devil; that I am, moment by moment, sucking joy and energy from the lives of those I love. That I am part of the wild extremism of our world: the floods, the raging fires scorching our very earth, filling the sky with ash and the smell of dead animals. I am the evil that means we now have leaders who make up their unique version of the world and the law. Who assume that they can do whatever they want. Who dismantle the hard-won connections we make between different communities. I am the force destroying the last tiny joys in the last days we may still live with pleasure in our hearts.

I don't want to face that. I want at least some doubt, some hope that this is schizophrenia rather than the bitter reality that means I pray, one day, to have the courage to leave this, to sign off from this living stuff, to leave the horror and responsibility behind.

Look at our, almost triumphant, appropriation of the Autistic Community's statements that they are neuro atypical – just different – and that society needs to adapt to that. I thrill to this and then clamp down when I hear my colleagues and friends saying those of us with psychosis or whatever it is, could learn a thing or two here. That this is just our difference; that the attempts to change us from who we are, are just plain old offensive. Why force our difference into some uncomfortable fit that means we might have to meet impossible standards and scrutiny from the rest of society?

I clamp down, just as I clamp down when I see adverts with smiley people being loving to each other, breathing the message that smiling and talking are all we need to do. Just as I do when I see my friends, with whom I have shared memories of what it was like in the old asylums. Being squeezed into short programs, after which they will be pronounced fit to use their new-found skills for living in this bright, bright world. Where, of course, it is possible to take responsibility, to break away from your pale dependence on your friends and workers and leave those decades of sadness by the side of the road. Knowing that next time you want to die, when the night is dark and your stomach filled with terrible, lonely, white anxiety, you now have the ability to overcome this by yourself. And if not, at least access to the advice that a nice warm bath or a brisk walk will break you out of the despair that consumes you.

As you can guess by now, I am also angry at the delight we feel when we say there are a multitude of different realities and ways of seeing the world and just who is the person who can have the arrogance to say that their reality is superior and more real than ours?

I get it! Just as my drunken student friends from nearly four decades ago would try to get their head round the idea that just because you can see the three legs of a dining room table, that doesn't mean it has a fourth leg or even that it is a dining room table.

It is amusing in a way but I am pretty certain that my dining room table is a dining room table.

And I am pretty certain that however much we try to bend it to something more positive, to see it in different ways, approach it in different ways, that mental illness is something dark and dangerous and most definitely not something to be celebrated.

I can no longer count the number of people I have known who have killed themselves, and I certainly cannot count the number of people I know who want to die.

We say it glibly: 'Want to die.' It is almost commonplace.

People might be doing what I am doing right now, which is looking out at the most beautiful wash of orange across a blue-black morning, outlining the mountains I am passing on the train. Knowing that this evening I will be with a loving group of different families, bound together by love, where the children will be running wild or snuggling into their mummies, upset by some chance remark. Where we will be drinking prosecco and contemplating the hot tub despite the storm that is forecast.

Some, like me, may be looking forward to walking Dash the dog, by the Clyde among the seaweed, the sea smell, the rich mud smell, the sound of the birds and the whistle of the Helensburgh train.

To leave this? This ordinary but wonderful life? I would, I think. I think one day I will and I so don't want to. This is so lovely.

The people we love, the things we do, the sights we see, the food we taste, the stories we create, are something we would leave because our distress and our illness can be so awful that we see no light, no sunrise, no snuggled children, or dogs to stroke, just the prospect of oblivion and freedom from memory and thought and pain and somehow we celebrate this?

Somehow this is just what we are and this should be respected?

I think back to my memories of my brother, shouting down the phone at me when I was looking forward to coming off my medication – "Do you not know that when you are in hospital, the whole family is waiting for that phone call that says, finally, you have died?"

And although this was the first time I had heard him shouting, it was also the first time I had heard his voice cracking with the pain of it all; that pain they too have suffered over these years.

There *is* something brutal about illness or whatever this experience is. I went for my tribunal recently, in which they decided whether to continue treating me. It was a life or death decision and I still have no idea what I wanted that decision to be.

The worst part of my life which I cannot explain to the professionals around me, because they say I am usually animated and articulate and engaged, is that I am dead, or maybe not that. I am not here.

I remember times in my life when I was truly vibrant and how ideas and conversation were always bubbling to the surface. I remember times when everything was so present; you could almost touch the colours of the sunrise, you could feel the wide, energy-filled connection from your heart to people and the world.

I remember when sometimes I lived. When I inhabited life.

Now I don't and it has been so many years, so many years. I am so weary of it. I still sit on a rock at Ardmore with Dash the dog at my feet and watch the oystercatchers fly low above the water. Or the heron, still by the shore or the curlews flying away, calling their lonely call, or the crows hopping sideways on the seaweed and I am delighted, but I am delighted as though I am hidden behind a screen. Everything is at one remove. I am half asleep, lost in a pale dream.

Wendy, my partner, still sometimes begs me to speak, says I am in my ultra-quiet zone again, and I do try. I look for words but nothing is there; nothing at all. This not being. The not being alive thing, it makes me despair sometimes.

I think of all those journeys when I am convinced people are moving seat because they know what I am, or those social gatherings where, though I am enjoying myself, I mutter insults at myself because I know these friends and family members secretly despise me.

I remember the sizzle of cigarettes on my skin, my flesh made tough by repeated dousing in boiling water. I remember the slick pain after razor blades have passed across my wrist and wee Charlotte's queries about how I got the scars and her mum's fear at how devasted she would be if she knew that, even now, I still consider my death would be a boon to the world.

Or those nights: the times with the red raw eyes because, night after night, you are up in the early hours and even the World Service won't drown out your battering thoughts.

And we would paint this differently? Repurpose it? Remodel it? Say to each other: "Stop making out this is some tragedy! Why not look at all the undoubted talents we have as a community, the joy we can bring to each other, the power of our hope and our desire to make the world a better place?"

We say: "Stop looking at what is wrong, stop concentrating on our deficits, on our terrible, terrible despair. Remind people that we can work, we can laugh and contribute and be of value, not only be of value, we are of value."

Yes, true of course! But me? I am also going to remember that although that 'Glad to be Mad' t-shirt was a wonderfully defiant act when I was young and naïve and, in some ways, innocent, that many of the people I knew in those days are no longer alive. Living became too difficult for them.

I want to remember them, not as atypical somethings, nor as oppressed people or any of that, but as people I cared for and who experienced illnesses the like of which you would never ever wish on anyone, and who did indeed smile and find different meanings to what they went through, but who suffered terribly, just as so many people I meet every day of my life continue to do so.

Naively, I want that to stop. I want to sit on that rock by the Clyde with Wendy and Dash the dog and really hear the seabirds, feel the wind, smell the salt air. Just once I want to turn to Wendy and say, "Do you really hear them? Do you feel this? I do!"

I want everyone I know to understand that void and feel that absence, and the joy connection would bring again. I want all these parcels of horror I have experienced and witnessed to be remembered and never glossed over with that 'Glad to be Mad' t-shirt I was once so proud of.

Three weeks ago, my mum asked for a proper hug before I caught the train home to Scotland. We hugged in the kitchen and then at the station there was a rare parking space, so we hugged again. She felt so thin; her optimism, for once, may have held a tug of uncertainty.

On the train a loud family talked about how they needed to get to the Isle of Man before travel was stopped, their luggage overflowing into the aisle, taking up spare seats.

And today. Now that we have had the children out of school for a couple of days, we walked round Ardmore. I kept trying to record the sea, the sound of the oystercatchers and curlews, the seaweed popping in the heat.

I walked up to the old manmade something – maybe once it was a harbour or maybe some weird fish trap – high blocks of stone, old wooden stakes. The mussel shells crunched under my feet. Dash the dog sniffed everywhere, tugged on his lead.

You, my love, got the children writing in chalk on stones. You got them to sing songs of the seashore; to stamp on the seaweed and carry lumps of wood to make their fort out of washed up polystyrene and twigs, decorated with shells and stones and flowers.

We all agreed it was a fine and lovely fort. I took photos. James, as is his way, put his face close to the camera so the shot was spoiled, but I got other ones I like.

We found frogspawn beside the path, thought of hatching the tadpoles at home.

At the point, looking out to the wrecked sugar boat, we again came across that massive, massive, washed up stack of wood and nails; some old pier come loose perhaps.

The gorse was yellow and smelling of coconut. You and the children clambered onto the wooden pier, James getting stuck halfway up. You all walked up and down, shouting out the numbers incised into the old wood, playing made up games, pretending to fall off.

Out to sea, the waves' own melody made this perfect; the gulls and the crows and the oystercatchers and the deep, deep, warm blue of the early spring made this especially beautiful; a treasured memory.

When we reached the bog, Charlotte nearly lost her boot in the mud. James cried at the scratch of the gorse we went through to escape the wet.

And now, back at home after the best, most perfect day of the year, the children say they miss their friends and we explain we are only allowed out once a day; that we are not allowed to visit other people.

I get ready to phone my mum, alone in her big house so soon after Dad died. You speak to your mum; try to convince her not to keep going out to the shops.

We sit later, confused, a bit lost.

April

2021—APRIL—WENDY—HAND IN HAND WITH SNOW FLURRIES FROM A CLOUDLESS SKY.

On our way to the reservoirs you delighted in reminding me just how off-kilter my memory was when thinking about the route we used to take to go to the wild garlic glen, which is also on the way to the reservoirs and somewhere we frequented, scant months ago. You mentioned how convinced I was yesterday that I knew the route; reminded me of interminable drives up tiny roads ending in hard-to-turn-back cul-de-sacs. I quite like being teased, especially as, without it, I am in danger of a pomposity overload.

We found the parking space, this time, found the path. Another sunny April day; the daffodils just beginning to fade. Just inside the gate to the field, through which the track runs, we found an old cart: green-rimmed wooden wheels, on its side, its seat parallel to the earth, yellow trim, the bed of it pointing into the ground in a scatter of rusty metal and decayed wood.

I had to take a photo; gathering in the memorabilia of our day to day, pausing just a second to think that this oddity might, and probably did, rattle along tracks with birdsong, conversation, laughter, the occasional stony-faced, silent quarrel. Trying to remember such things mean so much more than an Instagram mention.

Our conversation was light. I love the lightness you bring to life. And am still confused that you don't grump more and that, even when you are in a full on grump, seem unable to express it with any conviction. This would have been just as your UTI was slowly fading away but you were still tired, and just as your endo pain was flaring up again, making long walks a painful and weary experience despite the green grass, budding trees and occasional flower.

We passed a broken caravan, then a derelict house, piles of rubbish beside it. A paddock with nothing in it. A makeshift pen with chickens clucking. We paused to look at the remains of a cutting into the hillside. Then another derelict building which seemed to be some sort of very large, abandoned toilet block. The sort you might have found in the Victorian section of a once prosperous city. But then, it could have been some long-forgotten milking shed!

Dash the dog wandered along the edge of a ravine, much to your alarm, which was, maybe, justified, as he is very good at falling off things.

We never did find the reservoirs. We veered off track, climbed another steep hill through whin bushes and, when you declared yourself unfit and unsupplied with your inhaler, sat on rocks by a drystane dyke wall.

Dash sat himself down and stared, like us, down to the Gare Loch. A silver sparkle of bright water, studded with ships and yachts. Beyond that we could see to Gourock, on the other side of the Clyde, and Dunoon, beyond Roseneath. Not the slightest breath of wind, blue sky, no clouds, lots of sunshine.

We wondered about ticks, paused to greet another couple walking up our faint track, confirmed to them that we did not know where the reservoirs were either.

I was just settling to do some more daydreaming, maybe have a kiss or two, perhaps join in a conversation about I have no idea what, because such things seem to arrive like magic from your lips. I never have a clue what to say but do love the stories you tell; the thoughts you express, the opinions and meanders in your imagination you gift to me as a matter of course throughout the day.

Suddenly you said, "What time is your Zoom call?"

I replied that I had ages yet but that it was at three and you pointed out it was twenty to three, that we were up a hill and twenty minutes drive from home!

Walking downhill was so much quicker than our breathy struggle uphill!

As we walked it began to snow.

"What on earth is that?" we asked each other.

I thought there must be a fire nearby with lots of ash; you opted for dandruff!

We refused to believe snow can come from a cloudless sky but when the white specks landed on us and melted, we had to agree on the snow option.

I wish every day was like this: adventures to all sorts of places. In this case, a stunningly beautiful, almost post-apocalyptic landscape of hills and grass, bracken and woodland and abandoned buildings where we wittered, walked hand in hand with no particular end in sight. Where we teased and laughed and got muddy feet, stumbled through whin bushes, sat on moss-covered rocks, watched the tiny yachts below us, tacking up the water.

Maybe if we had more time, we would have taken advantage of the isolation to cuddle and kiss and caress, our eyes a little bright, our breath a little fast.

We walked back, hands swinging together, thinking about distant times when we had nothing to worry about, no demands, no need but to snuggle up and sleep for a while. But just then, we needed to be home in time to switch on the laptop, log on, say hello to distant people and hope the rush upstairs didn't betray my hurry.

2021—APRIL—MY JOURNAL

April has been that wonderful start to summer. I have been finding the smell of spring everywhere, of flowers and earth, the gorse and the daffodils. The birds are beginning to be very noisy in the mornings, I am beginning to wake, not from dark dreams or the noise of the world service, but because the sun is shining through the window.

Wendy is now recovered from her UTI and that evening with the ambulance is long gone. Her endo pain is still there, rustling away, making her tired and exhausted each month and each month astonished that it is painful; each month when she has recovered, sure that she must have been making it up.

I have been writing speeches and I have been writing articles and I have been learning a little bit more about photography at a course at Jean's Bothy, the mental health centre I go to. We have been off galivanting in gardens full of flowers. Wendy has been promised her jag because she is my carer and will get it in May, the day after my second jag. My mum has had hers already.

The last lockdown has eased and we have spent time with Peter and Sharon and David and Clare and the children, a blossoming of connection. Though, in the name of connection, Wendy accepted one too many drinks from Sharon and had to take to her bed instead of painting Charlotte's skirting boards as we had planned.

Colin, who I knew for many years, and who provided many quotes, much frustration and a lot of affection, turns out to have died just before Christmas, alone and left for some weeks until the police kicked the door down. Another person, Dianna, has also died after years in what seemed quite demeaning conditions. Debbie, a person I managed when I worked at HUG, and who was lovely, who I had fairly recently met to interview about her own experiences, got work in a nursing home. I had given her the reference for it. She posted about the lack of precautions they were taking over Covid and then she caught it and then she died. They would be my comrades, my somethings; there will be a tale in their deaths that I don't really want to politicise. I hope I can instead, remember them as lovely people.

My dad's birthday passed and I had some especially vivid dreams of him that night but I did not mention them on my evening call to my mum. Somehow, the overt display seemed a bit too needy and a bit too demanding of my mum to reciprocate with her own feelings. I did like it when Juliet put up a post to Dad on Facebook and mentioned the whisky she was drinking and a lighthouse, which I think is a reference to the poem she recited with the children at his funeral. His birthday made me remember the time, a few years ago, when I went to the vinery with Mum and Dad for his birthday meal, a lovely tender time, very quiet. I do not know if such things should be said but to me they are so important. I remember on that trip my mum saying she was fed up that Dad didn't acknowledge all she did, that he almost expected it and Dad saying how little he did with his life, that struggle to work out each other's new roles when they were both husband and wife as well as carer and patient.

Those last years, I find it hard to look at them – the times when the children were fractious and upset over Sandy's illness, the times when poor wee James could not quite accept my presence in the family and to be fair, neither could I. Wendy went to such efforts to show me that when I joined in and was silly that James was over the moon and delighted, tried to show me that the needs of a grown man and his insecurities were less than those of a little boy. But I did not know how to deal with that.

Those years! Sandy's cancer, my dad's Parkinson's, my uncertain settling with my new family, my worries about work and the reactions of people I would have called my peers, to it, has carried a toll.

It is only now that I really think I will remain here, that it won't go wrong. I won't get sacked at work or find myself suddenly packing my possessions, off to find a new place to live in again, alone...

Our dads are dead and that still sometimes surprises us. Frequently, we say how wonderful it was that they died before lockdown started, how awful that would have been. It would have been so bad for Sandy, on his own, getting weaker and weaker, without us to come in every day with the messages and conversation. I remember he reserved a week after his chemo to stay at home but after that, he really wanted to see family. I think not having that would have felt like a special torture and I am sure my dad would have been indignant about some of the restrictions and my mum even more exhausted than she had been getting.

I haven't been struck by grief or memory much at all this month. I am still reading my dad's memoir. I have just got to when he had set up Alan Morgan Yachts and had left the Air Force. It is a very strange and slightly alienating experience, reading about his life; we don't really feature at all! There are about ten sentences covering our childhood and our family and the rest is about his flying and his ocean racing and his cars and his business. I am tempted to be angry and then have to remind myself of different times and values. I still sometimes see posts on Facebook or Twitter, exhorting people to set goals and to strive for them, to achieve and achieve in the world of work and what passes for success.

I am sure that my dad did that, that he measured his life by the recognition he got and the achievements he made. I need to remember how bad he was at talking about emotion and love. That my parents are, and were, private people in these spheres of life. Maybe to write down how he felt about the people in his life would have been too difficult for him, or some crass breach of etiquette, but I had hoped to find something of what he thought of us all and what he remembered of his life with us and am sad that it does not appear in his own record of the memorable things of his life.

Still, I have part four left to read and maybe I will find some sort of illumination there.

Also, I have to be honest with myself too. It is hard to write about people, even harder to write about the people you love but may sometimes criticise in your mind. The bringing into the public of family and friends which seems natural to me, is dangerous and upsetting to others. Wendy has already said she does not want to read this book when it is published, as it will bring back too many memories that she would prefer to avoid. I need to remember that but also to remember that my approach to life is also similar to my dad's.

I gave up all expectation of being as good a stepfather as I would like to be, and lost my right to being a real father years ago. I doubt my ability to even be a friend or an acquaintance. Many of the people who make my life shine will not appear here. I do not write about work that much but I do the same as my dad did by writing about myself and in real life I have to remember what I do in reality.

The last three weeks I have been working three evenings of each week, a mixture of paid and voluntary work. I say family is important, that I love them dearly, but how often do I demonstrate that? I do not wake thinking, what can I do today to make my friends and family happy and entertained? I wake to tasks: making breakfast, emptying the dishwasher, walking in front of everyone with Dash when we all go to school; planning what I will do at work that day, hoping I will do something that means in its own way that I am recognised and praised for doing a good job. It is a pale way to look at life.

Sometimes I wonder at all these years striving for justice and the voice of people like me. I no longer know what justice would look like. I no longer have a vision of what would make the world better, and when I do, I quickly reprimand myself for my arrogance. I spoke to a young woman last night about what would make a difference and we went down the route of being listened to, being hugged and needed and valued. In the past, I have said such words so many times too, but when she was speaking, she reminded me of the power of that vision. How, when you are alone in a ward on a section and you have nothing to do, nothing to look forward to and feel dismissed by all the staff, how a smile and a sprinkling of belief in your worth can be transformative.

In my work nowadays, everything is about ideas, rights and voice and making a difference, and it pains me. Maybe we do make a difference but I think the biggest difference I have made in all these years of striving has been to go for a walk with someone who has no one to walk with. Drink coffee with someone who is wary of being in public. Find a way of praising someone in such a way that they won't burst into tears because moments of kindness are too hard to bear. It is those things that make the difference.

And where do they happen? Not in a report or even in a speech, not in an article or a Teams call. But in Charlotte's expression when Wendy decided we would get a new floor for her room, or Wendy being content to look after the rabbits for the next fifteen years or so, already knowing that, although they are Charlotte's, that as a ten-year-old she will want to occasionally cuddle them or read stories to them but only occasionally.

The sky was bright blue this morning; when the children cycled to school they were delighted with the world and the sunshine. Later, while Wendy was with Paula, I sat on a log on a beach with Dash and felt happier than I had in a long time; that pause, the hot sand, the clouds and the sun and now, now the rain has started and I doubt our plans of going out adventuring after school stops will come to fruition. That is what is important really.

A few feet away from me, the rooks are walking on the roof by the chimney. Wendy is finishing her work for the week downstairs. I am trying to think how to take a good photo that illustrates how much I love writing and reading. We might have fish and chips for tea.

And back to it again, listen to yourself and pay heed, Graham! Wendy and James giggling uncontrollably to the song and the dance they made up last night. Charlotte grinning from ear to ear when she was on James' Xbox last night. That is what it is all about.

I think my dad must have known that but I am uncertain. I hope he knew how much that last hand clasp and statement of love meant to me on my last visit to him, shortly before he died, and that that meant much more to me than the success he had and sometimes didn't have in his life.

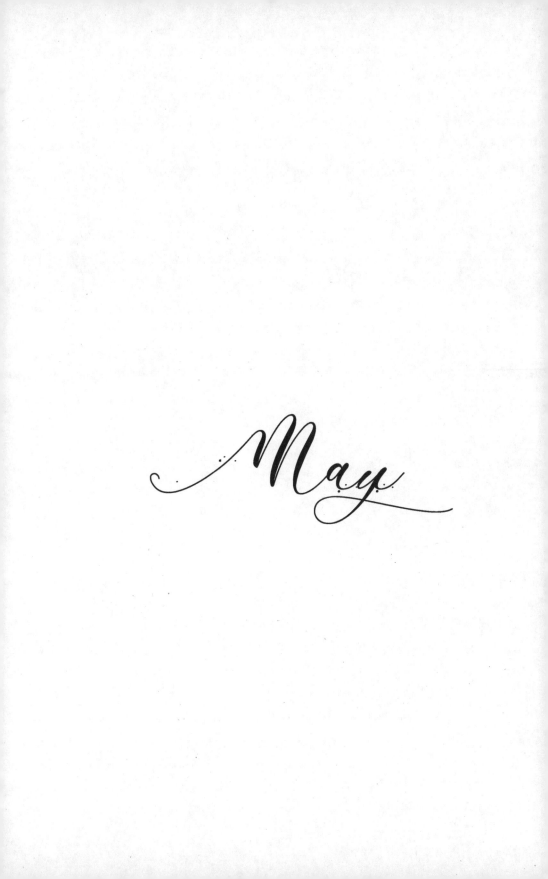

May

2021—MAY—WENDY—GLENARN IN SPRINGTIME

Those petals, pink-blushed, translucent from the sunshine, were stunning. Wendy and myself and the children had taken a break to walk in the Glenarn Gardens, with its streams and rhododendron and magnolia blossom; its daffodils and high trees, its view out over the Gare Loch.

I find it hard to understand how fortunate I am nowadays. Yesterday, I was talking to a friend who has mental health problems and who was once a CPN. She finished our call saying how refreshing it was to hear sense and perspective for once, and how wonderful my life had become in the last few years. She then joked about the wise advice madmen can give, which made us both laugh happily.

I do have a blessed life nowadays. I still worry that the children or Wendy will hear me when I am alone in the house and tell the silence around me that I want to die. I still wonder if I should, but that imperative is faint now. I hold on to life and find my memories of being under 'constant obs' in hospital, having to go to the toilet in front of the staff, hard to recognise as a reality anymore.

When I told my friend, the ex-CPN, that I was just lucky, she said, yes I was lucky but that I had worked hard to get to where I am now. I don't believe her, I think it is good fortune and the world around me.

As we continued our walk, Wendy talked, as she does; laughed. The children ran around in the damp, mossy grass. James decided he hated his lunch.

At the quiet bench James spoke loudly, in a stage whisper, and in between listening to the birdsong, we laughed together at our conduct. The woods smelt of earth and coolness, of damp freshness, and in patches were sweet with blossom.

It was a fairytale walk; this journey has turned into a fairytale life. I am no longer called 'Schizo', or 'Psycho'. I no longer anticipate chairs being thrown across the room at me or being spat at by someone who claims she loves me.

Instead, I walk with a brown fluffy labradoodle. Wee Charlotte never wastes a chance to tell me she loves me. James is almost funny when he tries to stop Wendy kissing me. I wake to the school run, I take breaks from Zoom and Teams to walk in places like Glenarn. Every day I find places and moments like this; hand in hand, scuffing the leaves; looking at the silver of the sea in the distance.

I am no longer hated and I am no longer alone. I make lunches for our stops at wee benches. I photograph the magnolia, photograph this miraculous family who have given me a reason to continue to walk and live and admire the leaves and flowers around me.

I am walking a springtime dream, and, to my astonishment, every moment is real.

2021—MAY—MY JOURNAL

A couple of weeks ago I got an email out of the blue from Gloucester Constabulary. A detective had found a letter I had written, about five years ago, to my old boarding school at Rendcomb. The letter was about a teacher who had acted inappropriately towards me and another child. He hadn't done anything particularly bad, just invited us into his tent on a climbing trip. The other boys had smirked and told us he always invited the youngest and prettiest children into his tent. What he did was not traumatic; he cuddled us too much, stroked us too much, caressed us too much until what had seemed funny became unpleasant and we had to repeatedly ask him to stop.

I was wary of him afterwards, stopped going on his climbing trips, stopped climbing altogether. Refused his invites to go to his room. The worst result of this was from the other boys at the school who called us poofs and gay, which in those days was an insult, but then they also called me a greasy dago and a wog, because of my mum's surname and my slightly darker than pure white skin. Children can be exceptionally cruel sometimes.

Anyway, I wrote to the school; it had nagged at me. I wondered if anyone else had been treated worse than we were; thought someone should know. They replied after a while saying that they had no knowledge of anything like that, but if I wanted to, I should go to the police. I didn't. Now I have these emails, someone wanting to talk to me as part of an ongoing investigation and I don't know what to think. Is it an investigation into this teacher? Is it about something else at the school? There were so many other unpleasant things that happened there. I will just have to wait and see.

I saw my sister a few days ago. I took her fiftieth birthday present across to Lochgoilhead and we talked and ate cheese toasties. We talked of family.

We walked in the hills above the loch, looking at the most beautiful views; walking among the trees, looking at moss and clover and streams and cliffs dripping with water, talking about Dad. Trying to work out what we think about it all.

Juliet is, I think, a bit confused at her lack of grief. She says Dad just slipped out of her life with hardly a ripple and I wonder if I feel the same. I haven't cried, I am rarely sad and yet somehow I think I am still very bewildered by it all.

When we got back to the village, Juliet said goodbye and that she would carry on walking with Frodo the dog. I, being unfit and needing to get back to cook the children's tea, descended into the village and felt really glad that Juliet often gets called to this village in her midwife role because there are a number of young families here. It makes me glad to see that she has these connections and that over the years will get to know more and more people in communities across Argyll.

Work is exceptionally busy just now. So many evening meetings and so much I don't know what. I wish I had never agreed to chair the compulsion group at the Scott Review. Our progress is painfully slow; the emotion is high and the belief that we can have debate and argument and reach conclusions, painfully misguided. Misguided because I have a few hours a week I can devote to this, and misguided because we need these shiny ideas of participation and co-production shaken down a bit. We have some lovely people who are so indignant that they were ever sectioned that anything that approaches the possibility this might continue in the future is anathema to them. We have wonderfully polite practitioners and officials with differing views, but how do we all speak out and challenge and give some sort of input when some people are seen as the source of all evil by some people and others as wilfully obstructive? Then you have me, who would normally never in a million years put himself forward to such a major project with so little time to reach conclusions.

I just remembered, I didn't put myself forward. I was asked. I know the issues but I don't know the evidence; I don't even know the Act in the way any of the practitioners at work do. I sense more and more that, although we have been given a purpose and should have one, that this group that could talk for month after month with little tangible result, perhaps because everyone knows it doesn't have the time, structure or capability to do what it is meant to do.

When I am not dealing with work stuff, it is other stuff like my nightly call to my mum. She talked recently about how she was delighted to have got rid of the big petrol lawnmower and how she would also like to get the barbeque taken away and the leaf blower that she was never able to use because it was so big. It is lovely that she is so pleased and that the garage will be free of clutter for when one of the grandchildren's possessions are put in it, but I ache with a foreboding of grief that I do not even want to contemplate when she lists all the things she is sure she will never use again because she is too old and frail to manage them. I do not like this knowledge.

*

I am back from a walk of sunshine and bright seas, with almost no wind. I had Wendy and Charlotte with me; an amble along Ardmore. The terns seem to have gone but the swallows are here and there are flowers everywhere, and the leaves – just so green, a fresh, light juicy green. Charlotte climbed trees, Dash got fixated by a particular scent, the sea was faintly rippled but that was it, just faint ripples and blueness. I am now upstairs while Wendy and Charlotte play with the rabbits and James plays on his Xbox. It is just a couple of days since I spoke with the detective and I am not entirely sure what I think. For some reason I really don't want to tell my mum about it, even though that teacher did very little that was truly damaging to me.

We spoke. I told my story. The detective confirmed that they already had evidence about that same teacher and that he would probably be prosecuted whether I gave evidence or not and that by now the teacher was extremely old. He is away to check that what happened to me was seen as criminal under the law, all those years ago. And then we need to find some way of me giving a statement remotely, and after that it seems like I will need to appear in court.

When I was talking to Wendy about it, I felt very hollow, a bit trembly. I don't know why. I now wish I had come forward all those years ago, maybe other people would not have suffered and yet, at the same time I feel a bit sorry for that teacher. He really must have very little life left to him; what a way to end his last years.

I am meant to be doing a drink diary at the moment. My CPN used to be an addictions nurse and is keen for me to reduce my drinking which is sort of great. I started off well but she wasn't around for my last jag and I seem to have lost my initial enthusiasm. Talking about mental illness,

I am not as sad as I was, even recently. I do not ache with my lack of emotion and my distance from people. I think it is maybe because it is the summer, the birds are all so busy; when I go out to walk Dash at night, I see cats and foxes and hedgehogs, the plants are growing in the garden; things are happening so much that I do not even have to try to distract myself from my thoughts. I am too busy for them. Or maybe it is because Wendy goes out of her way to check I am taking my antidepressants!

May seems to be a busy time. I got a renewal letter for my PIP, the other day. My initial panic was solved by the CAB person who told me that if nothing had changed, then I should say that and that there should not be a problem. I hope that is the case!

Wendy is now over the side effects of her jag. Initially she said she was fine and went out to have pizza in her friend's garage, while we ambled around at home. She had the most lovely time and drank more than she ever normally does but for the rest of the week has had a low grade headache and felt very tired. In contrast, I had no side effects with my second jag.

I worry about the complete easing of lockdown now that all these variants are arriving but do like the thought of Mum coming up, and our approaching holidays. Maybe that is hypocritical of me because I cannot for the life of me understand why we seem to be almost encouraged to fly off abroad whilst at the same time cautioned about it.

Wendy dreamt about Sandy the other night. I cannot remember the context but she woke up upset. I have lost my dreams of my dad; it is sleep, work, walk, tea and so on and of course the rooks in the trees who never shut up nowadays! I met my new boss and do not quite know what I think of her; there is too much work and too little time to reflect and feel comfortable in the trust needed to get to know a new person. I find that the things I do are not the things I would like to do. I would like to write and I would like to take photographs and learn how to do both better, but I only do such things in the scraps of the day, in between work and social media and Instagram stuff, late at night. I would like to spend more time just doing family stuff and I would like to learn to laugh. I would like to be at ease with myself and the world and to have the energy to think beyond set tramlines that make the route of my life so rigid.

It is a tiring month and this police stuff is preying on my mind. I would like to know what will happen next. I would like to know why I am tired and why I get irritable over silly little things that I would never normally be irritated about. Is it really the memories of those days of my childhood that the police have raised? I thought that I had long since settled in my mind that those times were maybe not the best but in no way traumatic and damaging. I really do not want to resurrect all those old resentments that I had assumed I had long, long ago laid to rest.

If I start blaming my dad all over again for nothing much at all, I will be so incredibly angry with myself.

2021—MAY—ALAN—FROM FLYING INTO THE DARKNESS OF THE HIGH SKY TO LEARNING THE VALUE OF FEEDING THE RABBITS…

This bit is about my dad and now I come to it, I have the most awful realisation that I never really knew my dad. Not really.

It dismays me slightly and makes me question my own role as a dad or stepdad, although we avoid that word in my new family.

I have finally finished my dad's memoir. I had hoped to gain an insight into him as a person and to his insights into us, his children, or my mum.

I didn't.

After thousands of words, I know a lot more about the working of Alan Morgan Yachts, Mystic Yachts and Trade Wind Yacht Charters.

I have read about weapons displays, the Israeli Airforce and RAF Akrotiri, of being scrambled to intercept Russian Bear Bombers and of boat shows and the design of lots of different, very beautiful yachts.

But the glimpses into my dad as a person are not there at all, except the poignant ending where he said he was a 'nearly person': nearly a very successful air force career, nearly a very successful businessman and nearly the producer of some of the most beautiful yachts in the world.

And even more sadly, the bit where he said he had loved what he did but at 78 (when he wrote his memoir) regretted that he had spent so little time with his family.

I have already said that my dad repeatedly told me in his later years, when alone with me, that he saw himself as an emotional cripple and then he would apologise. I mainly batted it away, said there was no need for apologies and that I loved him and was sorry for how I had treated him.

I so often compare myself to his faults, of which there were many, and I hope I can learn from those.

But comparing myself to my dad's faults, trying to learn from his mistakes? A good thing to do but it is far better and far harder for someone like me to celebrate his successes; the wonderful things he did and was, as a person.

I struggle there, but now realise that if my frequent dreams of my dad are to match the reality of my memories of him, I need to finally tear myself away from the insecurity and memory of resentment and learn the wonder of another person.

It is a hard thing to do. I am not perceptive. I am the opposite of a people person. I rarely gather great insights when I meet people. My knowledge of them is even more limited than the pitiful knowledge I have of myself.

Wendy thought Dad was wonderful. It will be her that will help me understand him better, just as she did when I first got to know her. She knew him for only a few years but I think she will help, not so that I can write this book, but so that I can learn to live in a world where I connect more with those important to me.

I first truly turned away from my dad when I was sixteen or seventeen. I now think he had the best of motives, but at the table for dinner, instead of casual chatter or laughter, he steered the conversation into debate and argument. I always ended up arguing with him, often with little idea of why. I found his skill at debate meant that I ended up arguing against what I first started saying. They were horrendous meals, so emotional and so humiliating and so exhausting. I think in his own way my dad was trying to help us all, me in particular. If we could hold our own, if we could question and look at situations logically and objectively then maybe this would hold us in good standing later in life. I think it was that.

I know, one late night, when he got both of us drunk, he told me that his intention was to shape me into the adult he thought I should be; that he had a plan worked out that would create the eventual character I would grow into. For me, those sort of thoughts and actions were unforgiveable. I was a young, very shy and very sensitive man trying to gain my own identity and independence and here was my dad deciding who and what I should be.

Now that I think about it, I wish I had had an ounce of the confidence that could have let me tease him about his ambitions. I wish I had been able to laugh at the silliness of it. But at the time it all seemed deadly serious. Those years and some of the events that happened afterwards meant that, by the time I was at university, I blamed my dad for a sizeable portion of the unhappiness I was experiencing. It meant that I made it clear when I attempted suicide that I held my dad responsible and refused to let him visit when I was in hospital. This carried on into much of my adulthood after that.

My dad's antipathy to my future wife, and her hatred of him, continued for decades. Any family get-together or holiday was an event where we expected things to go badly wrong. From furious, whispered, late night arguments with my ex-wife who said I was not defending her enough and that we should leave in the middle of the night and drive back to Scotland, to the traditional arguments of, I don't really know what: politics, vegetarianism, pacifism – the usual settings for what we tended to call 'debate'.

It was only when I left my wife that my world widened and I looked beyond my own blank hurt of years and years previously. I started to see my brother and his family, and my sister and hers. I began to call my parents regularly. And by doing so I learnt of so much that I had missed in the growing up of my nephews and nieces. Of the lives of my siblings and their partners. Sometimes I would find myself laughing, enjoying their company so much. There were nights sat by campfires with my sister's friends at parties in the Borders, where I was excused singing but did agree to read some of my poetry the next day. There were times lying on the coarse grass of the hillside above the seashore at Morecambe Bay, with my brother and his family, where life seemed pretty much perfect.

My parents started to come to me for their holidays once I lived alone. I forget the reason why they no longer went abroad, maybe my dad's bad back or his leg which he had shattered jumping down a yacht's companionway. I don't know what it was but they would come up, see my friends, we would cook together. I would walk the beach with my mum, with her delighted at the geese flying overhead. We would drive round the Highlands, stopping in hotels, taking photos.

Finally I met Wendy and she met my dad. I had got into such a rut of memory that I was slightly shocked and very surprised to find she thought he was wonderful. She said it was obvious that in the past he was pretty much a rogue, but that he had a mischievous glint to his eyes, he liked to laugh, he liked his wine, his whisky, a story or two. He liked a woman who could get him talking and laughing and he loved the fact that I was so obviously so happy with her. She liked that he was both shy and a little arrogant. Thought it funny when he tried to wind her up about Scottish Independence and all the other things that can make for awkward silences. She loved his past in his jet fighters and ocean races, his world of rich people and that sense that he had just a tiny touch of the James Bond to him.

It shames me that this was a revelation to me. I had never known I could be genuinely proud of my dad and really think of him as a kind and loving man; but a loving man ignorant about the bringing up of children and family; ignorant about emotion and vulnerability and tenderness. A product of the high octane culture of flying jet fighters in the sixties and seventies, the weird sexual politics of sailing horrendously expensive racing yachts with millionaires.

He knew no different. I think, in his time, being overly bound to family would have been seen as a mark of disgrace. In fact, in his memoir he talks about the efforts he and his fellow pilots went to free another pilot from the clutches of his wife, into a world of fast cars and drink and whatever it was men did in those days.

Now that I am so much older, I wonder at my own values, my own way of living. I fitted into my own world of expectations when I became an adult. In the world I lived, there were very defined ways of being that you would never admit to but would never cross.

I could quite easily say that my lifestyle, my friends and my career were a rejection of my dad's generation's lifestyle. It's pretty much taken for granted now, isn't it? I don't know if that is quite what it was, but I do know that I was not like my dad, and that I could never have fitted into his preferred image of what he might have wanted me to be.

I am shy. I have little wish to court danger, though I have often experienced it and engaged in activities like that. I am good at speaking but in company do not know how to. In fact, even in the privacy of my

107

home I can struggle to find the words I need to connect with people. I do not dance, sing, tell jokes, I don't tell long stories. I don't make a fuss in restaurants or in any situations, really. I love to think that I might be charismatic and some sort of leader but, if I am honest, this is just not me at all.

My sense is that Dad was once like that too, but that his energy and intelligence and drive to succeed meant that the shy, insecure person he once was, was discarded in the need to create something different in life. I am not jealous of that; it would have created far too much pressure for me.

It pains me, but try as I might, I cannot quite see the bright vigour of success as something to yearn for. I have never had a desire to drive fast, to race boats, to be impressed by money or possessions and if I am completely honest, I think that my dad's dramatic loss of testosterone when he got prostate cancer changed his character into someone so much more gentle and reflective; someone who no longer needed to dominate and conquer. Someone who could laugh at his own intelligence and conviction that he was always right. I think that once, many, many years ago I would have loved to have dazzled people with confidence and energy. I think I would have been overjoyed if I had thought I was sexy and attractive and that other people thought that. I might have been happier if I had been able to stand up to my ex-wife and make decisions on my own behalf. I would have been a lot happier if I had had the wit and vigour and spontaneity to be funny and vibrant in company.

But at the moment, I am happy with what I am. I am not even sure if I am jealous of my dad in that way. I do, I think, suffer fools gladly; I do like to stare at flowers in the spring and to amble aimlessly with no particular target in sight. To be honest, though, I am no longer jealous. I want to move further from my dad's world. I would like it if I downgraded my ambition even further. If I stopped writing articles for magazines, stopped trying to be the conscience of some of the people who work, oblivious of what they do in the world of mental health. I would like to stop yearning for a bigger salary, to stop gaining my validation from the reactions to the speeches I make and instead, remember that moment this morning when I asked James if his Cheerios were OK for breakfast and he said no, that he wanted pancakes. I wish that, instead of accepting he didn't really want them, that I had gone away and started cooking.

Now that is a very long journey from when I was hoping my dad suffered through his awareness of the pain I thought he caused me. I am pleased with that. I don't blame him any more and I'm also pretty certain that I was never really sure what I was blaming him for in the first place! And those times drinking beer in the garden, chasing after him in his buggy. Priceless.

2021—MAY—ME AND MY MENTAL HEALTH— WHAT IS NORMAL?

Over twenty years ago, a group of people I worked with got all fired up again with the need to challenge stigma and raise awareness about mental ill health.

We designed a series of exciting postcards to get across challenging or intriguing messages. One of these had a heading which was "What is normal?" and behind it, a picture of a white sheep in the middle of a flock of black sheep. We were all excited about the idea of the black sheep of the family and turning this on its head.

It was a truly wonderful project. We had thousands and thousands of different cards with different designs printed. We had holders to put them in for free collection in pubs, libraries, hospitals, cinemas, all sorts of places.

On the day of the launch, I was meant to give the opening talk at the press conference even though I was not the real lead for the project. I stood up, started talking and then slowly found my vision blurring, my words scattering and becoming slow; a white panic creeping into my stomach until my words stopped and a dear friend, and the true project lead, guided me to a seat and took over from me.

They were innocent days; a chance for the heat of the indignation at the rejection of difference, both perceived and real, to shine bright and for us to say,

"Come and talk to us, meet us, recognise our joint humanity, the kindness and the love we feel, just like you do. See our talents and our abilities, discover our backstories and realise there are all sorts of different ways of perceiving us and most of them are good."

I loved those days; they were so busy and so successful. For years afterwards I would come across people who had saved those cards and put them in their office or on their fridge.

In those days we were speaking at conferences or in schools; asking schoolchildren to draw their idea of what a person with schizophrenia looked like and when they had drawn a wild man with fangs for teeth, dripping blood, we revelled in the astonishment and interest of the children when we revealed that that was my diagnosis and that we are really pretty normal after all. We told our stories to the people who detained us. We read poetry, created exhibitions, and central to all of it was: *We may be different but we are also just like you, we are the people who you might become; we are your brothers, sisters, lovers, children and there really is nothing to be wary of.*

Now, many, many years later and after many more times in hospital on a section, I wonder.

I no longer feel normal in a slightly odd but maybe slightly lovely way. I no longer think I am just like everyone else and I no longer want to celebrate my difference.

Nearing my sixtieth birthday, I am weary and although my life is better than it has ever been before, I realise that it is scattered with pain and the knowledge of a difference that now, at last, I realise I wish was not a part of me and never had been.

I used to laugh at how my well off parents had wanted a life for me similar to their own, perhaps: middle class, married with children, a nice big house, a good job, dinner parties and safe conversations; skiing, sailing, rosy smiles, good schools, and I said that the life I had led instead was so different and so much better than that.

I know we should be proud of our difference, but I am not.

I am not in the slightest pleased with the memory that at my first suicide attempt my little sister just did not understand, had her certainty and hope and pleasure ripped out of her very young and very safe life, or that my mother, who had always been so full of smiles and laughter, took to taking long walks in the hills, leaving whoever was at home to make the dinners she no longer thought about, or how my dad would get drunk, get me drunk too and when we were well and truly drunk, reach out for a sentimental hug he wouldn't dare to try sober. Try it even though he knew I blamed him for my pain and that I would finish the night accusing him of I do not quite remember what anymore.

I am not at all comfortable with my memories. Of my devastated marriage, my son I no longer see, my scars, my times on constant observations, learning I was frightening my neighbour's children with my behaviour.

I don't care if this is not of my making, that this is an illness that I cannot control and shouldn't be blamed for, it is still a part of me; a bit of who I am.

When my partner begs me to speak because I have no words and spend most of my time at home almost mute, because the pretence of charm I have at work is too painful and exhausting to carry on at home or, when I am in company, I smile fit to burst but haven't a clue how to join in the conversation. I flush with the shame at what people think of awkward, inarticulate me.

It is all very well to say we need to accept and live with difference, but look at the last couple of weeks. For those two weeks I have had the best time in years; somehow that echo chamber where I have no emotion, where my life is more a smear of a life than something real, where my gaze is blurred and my imagination crawls at such a pace that I cannot connect with the vibrancy of those around me; that went. For days I have been connected with myself and my emotions. Being unreal, dead almost, has fallen from me.

Why! One day I found myself gargling a tune in a game with the children and laughed so much I spluttered water all over the table and, to my astonishment, realised that this was the first time in I don't know how many years, that I had laughed in such a way that I was really laughing instead of going through the motions.

It breaks my heart that that has been my life and that I have not been able to *be* in the way I wish I could have been for all those I love.

I feel so much for those I love and who somehow love me, that, for most of the time, they are dealing with a facsimile of me and when they aren't, they are dealing with someone with bewildering beliefs that could lead to my death and the untold trauma that would do to the children.

This is something to accept? To be proud of? This is the bright reality of the *"What is normal?"* postcards?

No! I don't want that and neither do I like the "Dare to be you" adverts. I am slowly opening my eyes to the playgrounds the children inhabit; slowly realising that, for all our ideals, that children like to fit in, like convention, find some forms of difference frightening. In fact, so frightening that the weird children, like I was, find themselves on the outskirts: never invited to parties, never in the middle of excited games in the playground, instead crouched, alone, in corners, staring at the ground, waiting for the day someone finds some label for them and moves them even further from the norm.

I am just like my parents now. I hope that Wendy's children always have friends, have people who want to speak to them, are not talked about in that 'other' way – I don't want them to grow up to find joy in a new set of postcards that painfully say that, despite our oddity, we are still, in some strange way, loveable.

I don't want anyone to experience that.

I stamp my foot! In desperation I say:

"Stop distress, stop pain, stop the terrible behaviour we can end up displaying when we have been excluded, abused and exploited. Stop sadness, stop our instinctive need to avoid sadness and tears and anger and weird words. Make the world one of flowers and love and compassion."

As if!

I know my dim and distant self had the right idea; that the acceptance of difference is what we need, but my difference is sometimes unacceptable to me and sometimes to others and yes, of course I know there is no such thing as normal, but how I yearn to be normal; to be like how I imagine other people are.

I would like to trust men. I would like to know how to party. I would like to know how to sleep through the night. To know how to play with the children. If I could know that I wasn't responsible for every tragedy in the world, if I could stop drinking, if I could speak to the school mums at the school gates and know when to not share my most intimate thoughts, if I could play golf, think of things for us to do. If, if, if…

I hate, almost beyond expression, being different. I want to walk down the street and recognise my neighbours. I want to wander downstairs and dance with the joy of being with my new family and not think I am the cause of their suffering. I would like to live for one day at least without wanting to die. One day at least when I can guarantee that my laugh will be my own.

Maybe it is too much to ask, but can I live that dream where I never needed to plead for my acceptance and the acceptance of people like me? Where I have never had to try to find some way of me accepting me?

Where life just *is*: you live it, love your family and friends and never for a moment doubt your right to it or the certainty of your journey?

It is only now that I realise just what we were saying when we were saying, *"What is normal?"*

We were not saying, *"Stop rejecting us. After all, we are just like you. We are as full of fun and laughter and talent as anyone else you meet."*

No. We were saying, *"We are not normal. We are often not pleasant. Our lives can cause untold pain to you. Our pain often causes us untold pain. We can be so disgusted by ourselves that we rip chunks out of ourselves, and rip your hearts with our lacerating anger at the world we live in. You need to deal with this because this is what the world is really like for so many of us. You need to accept us: warts, delusions, anxiety and all, even when that harms the certainty of your own lives."*

To be honest, I am not sure I can accept that either; I am not brave enough. I really do think the world should be meadows of daisies that we all dance among until we curl up to sleep in the orange blossom-scented warmth of a summer evening and wake in the morning, ready to stretch our arms out to dance some more, maybe sit by a stream; play some music…

That is the life I want. I don't want reality or normality at all.

2019—MAY—SANDY—THE AFTERMATH

Wendy had expected to be in floods of tears all the time after her dad died and yet she wasn't. She needed about two months off work, as did Peter, but mainly it was because she was so exhausted, just physically shattered.

We didn't know that grief could take this form. In some ways Wendy felt that she had done her grieving as she witnessed her dad's long journey to death in those months and months of worsening health. Those times when her heart broke when her dad was so down he couldn't crack a smile. That time when he was so weak he collapsed on the steps in front of the house in front of the children; the sepsis, the new cancer, the emergency operation; those exhausting weeks of hospital visits. The time he said it would be his last birthday with the children when he took them all to Build a Bear for their birthday.

It all ripped her to pieces and yet somehow she remained a vibrant and loving mother and partner.

The one thing she did not like was the need so many people had to say, "Stay strong."

She resented that – didn't like the pressure to cope, the judgement it implied if you could not stay strong.

She also found the occasional conversations with people who had known her dad and whose kind words made her cry, difficult. She hated crying so much. She is like her dad in that way. I remember when her dad was in hospital on that last day; she was so relieved no one reached out to hold his hand. She said he loved family more than anything but hated hugs, hand holding, that sort of thing; overt displays of emotion.

I am glad I know her enough that I knew this might be the case as I was very tempted in those final hours, to just hold Sandy's hand.

She much prefers a dark and bitter joke that brings lightness and relief to the gushing of feelings, but at times in the last few months she has done something with me or the children and thought, "I must tell Dad that," and then remembered she cannot tell him. And at these times, tears can overtake her and I so wish to cuddle up to her, to take away that pain with my own hugs and she so often has to say that I am doing that for myself as, at such times, she wants to be left in her own space.

And there have been long, long nights.

I think this is where she can be truest to her thoughts and feelings, where she is alone and does not have to look after anyone, think of anything other than what she wants to think about.

Sometimes she wants cuddles at these times, but rarely. Respecting this is hard. Knowing this is her journey and that I will probably never understand it, and at the same time feeling relief when she is making plans; working out where we will live when we are older, how we will look after a new dog when Dash is old and I am decrepit. I am so glad I am still a part of this unique family.

Charlotte was the most overtly affected by her papa's death. She didn't go to school for a week and, for a few months, was incredibly badly behaved at home. Even Wendy's patience was tested when she was deliberately driving us up the wall; making completely impossible demands, feeling extreme emotion. Yet Wendy, after the initial irritation, her momentary wish to send Charlotte to her room for the next two weeks with not even bread or water, would always pause and consider and eventually manage to get Charlotte talking.

Each time, when alone and cuddled up with her mum, and calmer, she would burst into tears and just say she was missing her papa. That missing her papa made her behave as badly as she could and she did not know why and could not stop herself.

She still does it nowadays but less often. She sleeps in her mum's bed now, frightened of monsters, needing cuddled and protected.

James seems to have taken it in his stride but sometimes we get glimpses. He shuts away emotion but also often climbs up to his mum's bed too, does the typical 8-year-old boy thing – avoids anything resembling a hug at the schoolgates and yet cuddles up with his mum to witter and laugh and confide every night, when they are alone and it is just him and his mum.

He needs his mum. He is very open about the fact that he is really jealous of the affection Wendy gives me. He tries to avoid sitting on the same sofa as me; often won't take a drink or food if I have made it or handed it to him, and I have grown to see that this doesn't matter too much, that sometimes he needs a baddy to blame when he does not know how to make sense of things.

Both the children are always wanting their mum, squabbling over who is closest to her, squabbling about who has the greatest right to sit next to her.

Everyone was affected and still is. Wendy sometimes has a very, very difficult working life and this, combined with Sandy's death and the return of her endometriosis, means she is still often totally exhausted, seeking her bed and her own company. Eating and eating chocolate and crisps to find glimpses of pleasure while I am much less affected but drink far more than even I used to and find it hard to contemplate cutting down on the whisky.

Somehow, after Sandy died, a night without a drink became unheard of. It helped me to sleep and relax or at least it seemed to, even though I know it doesn't.

It helped me with my silence which is sometimes deafening in the irritation and awkwardness it causes.

And Dash? He has been indispensable. When Charlotte is too angry to get a hug from a human, she cuddles up to Dash the dog. James has overcome his initial flapping from the top of the couch at Dash's bounciness and now he adores him, rushes to see him in the morning and after school.

And Wendy? He is someone that Wendy can pour her love into and who will love and adore her in turn with no pressure, no demands.

I am his main walker and though I need less than everyone else in the wake of Sandy's death, those walks!

Today I had a gale on my face, the cry of seagulls and the roar of the wind in the trees, the crash of waves on the beach, the smell of the sea and the seaweed on the shore and that buffet and the patter of tiny drops of spray thrown at me by the wind.

I adore those times. I am so delighted that Dash the dog gets me out walking every day, easing my muscles, easing my mind, letting my harsh thoughts settle.

Sometimes I think it is me who has gained most from Dash; the walks, the feel of his head on my feet late at night when I have gone to bed. How he positions himself, as far as is possible, midway between all of us if we are in different rooms. Yes, Dash brings joy, almost as much joy as if we had had a baby but with none of the exhaustion.

*

The last few months have been very practical. I didn't realise they would be so organised. They have been a time of sorting and settling.

Initially, Wendy zoomed around with Peter, getting death certificates and funerals sorted, wills and pensions.

For Wendy and Peter these last few months seemed very healing in a strange way, just the sorting out of a life together. We spent a lot of time sorting the house, going to barbeques at his and Sharon's, doing this and that together. Making what are often nowadays very fractured families, with lots of different dads and mums, into a makeshift but loving extended family.

The first time we walked through the door into Sandy's house after he died was strange.

Just the silence; realising how messy our houses can get and realising sadly, just how few of our possessions have any value to other people. Looking at the clothes Sandy used to wear every day and thinking many of them were no use even for charity shops. Looking at all the computers and finding out most of them were too old to have any value at all.

It was mainly Wendy and Peter who sorted the house, but I helped when I could, emptying the conservatory, which had become more like a storeroom, into the skip; realising that it was a lovely room.

Piling shoes and jackets into bags, finding box after box after box of military magazines that went straight into the skip too.

Cleaning the kitchen of years of stains and grease; sorting the possessions into the tiny pile that family wanted to keep.

Looking at a diary of Sandy's which would have been the one thing I would have wanted to keep, but when Wendy took a quick look inside, at his private and very sad thoughts, realising that neither Peter nor Wendy wanted these words to symbolise the father they had loved, that book also going to the tip.

Then the library. Hundreds of books about ships and military history. Initially thinking it best to sell them on eBay. Then getting a book dealer along, who took a few boxfuls, then learning about Ziffit. Wendy and Peter spending hour after hour, talking to each other while scanning the codes of CDs and books and stacking them in cardboard boxes for collection.

Emptying the drawers and cupboards, realising we did not need more plates or pots and pans. Realising that some of the things we thought would be useful would be just constant reminders of death. All of them going either to the charity shops, the skip or the dump.

Slowly the house emptied.

Wendy made it pretty for selling, putting in cushions, painting the occasional wall, buying the occasional house plant until, after maybe three months, it was ready to put on the market.

The garden had been mowed, the balls from next door's children thrown back over the fence.

The tins of oil, the pots of paint, the wallpaper and car polish; all this stuff had gone and Sandy's beloved Mazda was away to Gary the mechanic, who Sandy had always promised it to. He always felt he would appreciate it and care for it in a way we wouldn't.

The house sold within the week. The last bits of furniture went to the charity shops, the last bits of junk got picked up. Harvey, Sandy's friend, was given the last of the books when he came up from Newcastle to visit, taken to lunch, nattered with. And then there was that point at which we were saying goodbye to the neighbours, saying we wouldn't be back, would most likely not see them again.

A strange, almost lonely feeling.

As usual, life carries on. I am slightly sad that I went back to see Sandy after he died, as the vision I have of him when I see him in my mind, is of his dead body. I would prefer to see him on those occasions when Peter and Wendy were both round, being silly, or when he was in Barca's feeling happy with us and the children, talking about the food, or at the place where he took us to watch the salmon jumping, only to see nothing but having a lovely time anyway. Wendy, anxious the children would fall in the peat brown water; Sandy talking about how his dad had taken him there when he was a child and how he hadn't seen the salmon that time either, but had always remembered it.

Maybe a better memory would be that grin of his when he pressed down the accelerator of his car and it shot forward, screeching; that relief from the tension, which I promised not to tell Wendy about or maybe not even that, his expression at Christmas when he was still well enough to enjoy his food, well enough to put a bright mask over his eyes and pose for photos in the restaurant.

June

2021—JUNE—WENDY—THE SCHOOL RUN

Life nowadays is mainly about walks; we have little else to do. Wendy is not the most walky of people; she does not tend to meet people to go for a walk and a talk where you can say things without quite looking at them. She prefers to be present, if you know what I mean. Talking in a café or sitting in a garden, eating cake and wittering with a friend.

We held hands today, walking home after dropping the children at school. Wendy said she had nothing she had to do at work today and that it would be hard to make herself work. As we walked and nattered, she did her usual idle picking at the leaves from the bushes overhanging the road. She nipped at a piece of moss from a wall which came free in a long, long, straggly length which she carried for a while before finding another wall to place it on, patting it tenderly in place.

In the house, we had tea and coffee, watched the birds at the bird feeders. Wendy announced that if the seeds attracted rats we would need to move house; talked about how wee Charlotte seemed happier now that she had got the courage to talk to her teacher about another girl who was being cruel to her; mentioned that James was much more friendly to me nowadays and often spontaneously barked, "Woof Woof" in thanks when I brought him his meals.

We talked about how people make it clear that they don't want another person in their company; how Lewis would have just said, "Why are you following me around, when I just moved away from you?"

And how James would just ignore the person completely until they got embarrassed, and yet how Charlotte would be embarrassed and awkward and not able to be overtly rude. We mused on it.

I mused on how Wendy can laugh one moment, be serious the next; make fun of life and treasure it too.

I ran out of words. Wendy decided she better start work. Said she was so glad that Clare likes to work with the telly on in the same room; said that people were snobby when they thought having the telly on was naff while having the radio or music on was almost seen as sophisticated.

These are the sorts of days I love.

2021—JUNE—MY JOURNAL

This month has passed me by somehow. I tend to think I can see a theme or a structure to a month and of all months, this one should have a theme, but it feels bitty. If I look back at it, I cannot see the story or the shape I might make out of it.

I no longer see my dad in my dreams and am very cross about this. I thought I was getting to know him there, but that memoir sent me, I think, into a hissy fit and now I don't want to see him and yet, of course I do. I see other people, though. I met Calum, my son, not long ago and then I met Betty, my mother-in-law who died some years ago. We were tidying up the wreckage after a whirlwind had played havoc in a superstore. I had this enormous bag of rubbish, I mean huge! Bigger than me. I turned it upside down but in exactly the wrong way and all the rubbish fell out again, all over the floor, Betty was very kind in helping me work out how to clear it up, just a wonderful presence, though I am not too sure we did actually tidy it away. Even I can sort of get its message, I think.

We visited my ex-sisters-in-law just last week, such a hot day! We had been to visit Kate, my ex-boss, in her garden for an open garden event. Lovely, especially when Maruska, her wife, introduced the children to the frogs in the pond. After our wander there, we found ourselves in Gill's garden where she tried to deal with the horror of having three dogs prowling round her pristine house and peeing on her garden furniture and we tried to keep Dash from Milk, the Rottweiler, who developed a dislike of Dash when both dogs took an indecent interest in Raven the girl, not so puppy, puppy anymore.

We ate rolls and cakes and nattered. I mainly talked with Gill, who reminded me again about how much her mum had liked me and told me how fed up her mum had got with my ex-wife in the last months she had to live, and also repeated the story about how liberated the sisters had felt when they finally realised that they did not like my ex-wife or her sister and wanted free of their control. We giggled about that first time I met up with them again, when everyone had exit routes and I had instructions for what to do in case anyone who knew us all, and might tell the other sisters if they saw us eating together. It is, as she said, sad that middle-aged people can be so frightened of other family members. It was lovely to see everyone again – sisters-in-law, husbands/partners, nieces and boyfriends, and of course, the dogs.

My policeman has been back in touch to say he has enough information to write a statement from me which he will check with me in a few days time and get me to sign it somehow.

Perhaps it is this that makes me cross with my dad and surrounded by my dreams. I had thought the detritus of the past was happily settled but I have found myself cast back into memories of childhood and that infuriates me because I know it wasn't that bad, but I have a story in my mind that it was. It prompted me to write a blog piece on privilege and the experience of public school, perhaps the only one that has caused a reaction when I posted it and it led to one of those mortifying episodes of self pity.

I became immersed in memory, much of it bitter, and I just went on and on to Wendy about my wish to be rid of this schizophrenia stuff, to be rid of the past, to, to, to… Until she got fed up because there is the need to speak, but the desire to wallow in the dirt of it all can be so off-putting. She also got fed up because I had stopped taking my antidepressants and, alongside my CPN, thought that explained the place I found myself in.

All that bitterness from me; it was this time, not so long ago, that Sandy was sitting silent in the Masala Twist restaurant, his chemo overtaking him, just sitting there, head in hands, not eating, until he could decently leave us all and go home to bed. That is something to remember. He didn't complain or whinge or anything like that which I am so inclined to do. When he could, he was with us, when he couldn't, he tended to stay at home.

My mum came up, a long process. She got picked up by Richard and taken to Tunstall for a week, where she stayed with the family. Then Wendy and I went down on the Saturday and arrived early afternoon. We had a late afternoon walk, down by the river where the cows are, with the pool the otters sometimes swim in. I loved the evening with everyone. Richard has made a stand for his pizza oven and the evening was a feast of pizza. More delicious than I knew pizza could possibly be.

It was lovely having my mum with us. We seemed to spend most of our time in gardens, surrounded by fragrance and massive blooms of flowers. Flowers and walks and nattering of a sort. It is strange seeing how tiny Mum is, and thin, and how she struggles on rough ground because she cannot see quite well enough to place her feet with certainty. My mum would protest at the 'tiny' label with justification, she is tall and, for her age, a hundred times more fit and resilient than me but somehow she seems tinier than I remember from childhood and so, for some reason, I use that word. The number of times she told me I was lazy, though! I suppose, compared to her, I am. She gets more and more frustrated if there is nothing constructive for her to do other than relax and talk, always has to do stuff and my determination to 'treat' her maybe has the opposite effect.

I think perhaps, despite knowing that there really is no legacy of trauma from my childhood, I do resent the need I have to achieve and succeed; to get to the top of the hill, cook the perfect meal, write the best speech.

Wendy has taught me the wonder of not having to do stuff, the joy I am very slowly learning, about having fun with the people I am with, the things I do. The importance of relationships and caring for people when so much of my life is bound up with thinking people hate me and that my work is really no good at all. I can find it hard to relax and accept that some people do treasure me.

I dropped Mum at Oban for her cruise. Such an exciting thing to do. I still don't really know where she went but do know that the weather was bad for the week she was there and that Richard and Kathryn had similar bad weather for their sailing holiday in the same area, which was marred even more when Kathryn got a kidney infection and had to spent some days on a drip in Oban Hospital.

We had our first proper meal of the end of lockdown with Peter, Sharon, Clare, David and all the children. I was tired because I had driven to and from Oban already and was then driving to Bearsden and in great need of a drink by the time we were settled at Peter and Sharon's house after our meal. Wendy has been declared an honorary sister by Clare and Sharon and is delighted. I think the feeling is mutual.

We have mixed much more, recently. Like when we met up with Juliet's family after she had picked up Mum at the end of the cruise. It is lovely to see all the children, to wander besides the lochside, but I worry about Covid variants and the fact that Wendy has still only had one jag. I tend to wish we would avoid contact and hugs but maybe we just need to get used to this level of risk.

I still don't know why I feel unsettled with this month. I think it is because I hate confrontation and hate to cause offence. I criticised a paper someone wrote a few days ago and the author took offence and ignored my criticism, and then a person I was talking to said she had to take the day off sick, mid sentence. I still think my behaviour caused her to go off sick but when I checked my emails with someone else, they said that what I had said was constructive and helpful and later, someone else confirmed that my main criticism of that paper was spot on, but still I feel I am blundering around causing harm wherever I go. The reassurance that others give me about my perspective and skill and behaviour does not reassure me. It makes me anxious about work. That pit of the stomach feeling when I contemplate work tomorrow shouldn't be there. All I have to do is to learn how to manage some sort of secure platform to speak to people in a secure hospital but the worry about messing it up will make me wake early and distract me from the sunshine and the wind of this lovely Sunday.

Wouldn't it be wonderful not to have to work? To step back from this striving, this changing the world stuff. I wish I could have the sort of life where I can see the important things, like laughing when Wendy climbs onto a chair and announces she has suddenly grown two feet taller, or just having the energy to talk and to relax; having the possibility of enjoying the wonderful life that I am in. Not looking at Twitter and getting irritated, not wondering if someone's barbed comments on social media are aimed at me, not worrying that I don't work enough when I know I work way more than my hours. It would be so good not to worry, so good not to feel exhausted all the time.

JUNE—2019—THIS GETTING OLDER THING— THESE CONSTANT EMERGENCIES

This time last year was probably one of the worst of months of my life.

I started off in the Highlands on a work trip I had been really looking forward to, as I would also be meeting many old friends and acquaintances, but in the middle of a meeting I got a call from my brother saying my dad had had a pulmonary embolism and then a heart attack.

I didn't quite understand the significance of this until Richard said I needed to come down but there was no need to hurry, the unstated bit being that Dad would almost certainly be dead by the time I arrived. He wasn't; he was in critical care and in fine form and delighted to see us and then in high dependency and then on a normal ward.

From the moment he regained consciousness, he insisted he should go home. He was incontinent, unable to get out of bed and often his conversation made very little sense but maybe that spirit of independence and that slightly arrogant self-belief and confidence that he would manage, is somehow something to do with how he carried on for so much longer.

He did eventually get home. Work let me work from England for a few weeks so that Mum had support and company and then I went back home to Wendy.

However, just now, now that I am with Mum and Dad again, I am a bit angry at the health service. Dad was meant to get physio within a couple of weeks of getting home, but it took over nine months. If physio had happened sooner, he might have had more of a chance to adapt to his condition and work more with it. Maybe not, but it feels that way.

And Mum is exhausted. Her eyes are always red and hollowed from whatever all this eye stuff is and she is so bad at telling us of her disabilities. I am still shocked that just a few months ago she admitted that she can only hear us with the aid of a hearing aid, and that she has had one for years and has never felt the need to let us know about this.

I felt for them so much and felt guilty that I have done so little, apart from the visits and the phone calls.

I do not fully appreciate Mum's courage and determination; her cleaning up after Dad, her washing his soiled clothes, keeping the house clean, her constant work with the church and her friendship with all the people who live near her, her volunteering with the Samaritans all these years, swimming almost every day, still going in the sea in the summer.

131

Her determination to include Dad in the community, even though he has retreated, says less and less, does less and less, and saddest of all, seems to have lost the ability to thank her, to let her know how much she means to him.

After so many decades, I think it must be hard, this shift; the fact that for so long Dad decided, did, ordered. Was The One and now Mum's constant support is the most important thing.

To be totally honest, I now dread old age. There was a time, a couple of years ago, when almost every time I phoned home, I would hear that yet another close friend of theirs had died. That they were back from a funeral, sending a condolence card.

How do you cope with the fact that, when you are old and your sight is bad and you can hardly walk, that the people who make your life the good life it is, are also busy dying?

It seems to me worse than a war zone. There is no hope of victory, there will be no happy outcome. Eventually Dad's Parkinson's will kill him. He will probably end up in a care home. He will no longer be able to walk, to speak, to string a sentence together, and slowly Mum will probably go blind with her glaucoma, will hear less, will no longer be able to drive or go on her walks down to the church or across to the Samaritans in Eastbourne.

I hate it. They have so much humour, so much dignity. They smile at life and yet it will get harder and harder. Why are old people not celebrated for what they face? Why are they not our heroes? Surely the fact that my mum is always being positive, always doing and making light, should be acknowledged? Isn't the fact that, although Dad is resigned to his disability, is probably a bit or a lot depressed, that he can still make jokes about it; isn't that incredible?

I remember that time we went on a journey to a National Trust place and how, after some time, Mum told Dad he was giving me the wrong directions and how it became obvious that we knew he had no idea where he was going but were too embarrassed to say so. I carried on following his directions and he got quieter and quieter until suddenly Mum saw another completely different National Trust Place and said, "Let's go there instead."

Dad agreed to this with considerable relief but he was able to joke about his declining navigation skills that evening and make us laugh. It seems to me, to keep dignity and humour in the face of these things deserves medals and TV programmes and yet instead, I think we tend to look at older people with a degree of distaste.

There are so many times when I speak to Dad on a Sunday when we have had to make a joke about how bad we are at speaking to each other and that maybe it would be better to put the phone down or speak to Mum instead, and I am so bad at asking the wrong questions.

I will ask: who won the tennis? And he will go silent and ponder and eventually we will agree that someone won the tennis but it doesn't matter who, or I will ask him about the reading he does, which he loves so much, and then he confesses that he finds it a trial because after a few pages he has completely forgotten what he was reading about.

Why do I always phone on a Sunday after they have eaten their tea? Why do I never think, I would love to speak to Mum and Dad and just pick up the phone? I both do and do not understand this. I know the few times I have done that they have been almost as shocked as me.

And why, when I was in Highland enjoying myself, getting ready for meetings and events and I heard Dad was about to die, was I able to be calm?

How was I able to get in my car, sure that when I got back to Wendy, I would hear that Dad was dead but there were no tears, no problems driving, a hollow stomach but that was about all? And how, after that miraculous recovery, did I think to myself in secret and say to Wendy in private that it may have been better if he had died? If, in an instant, he was not there. He would have felt no pain and now he has this torturous process to live through and still he laughs, still he shows something special: how could I have thought that?

I have so much to learn from my mum and dad, from Wendy and her dad, from Peter and Sharon, from so many people.

Just the simple acceptance of love is so simple and so important; not the need to prove you are loved or the need to know you are loved in turn, no grand statements that mark us out as loved or loving. Just the knowledge that love can be a quiet thing, and stronger for all that.

Wendy and her dad had a sort of horror of hugging each other. It wasn't done much in her family but you can see her love for her dad and her family in everything she did.

Here is where her community, her friends and family live. Why would she ever leave such a place? Leave her family alone? What conceivable reason could there be for that?

I see that now. When I left home, travelling almost as far away from home as I could manage, and being encouraged in that, that maybe this need for us to cut our strings with family, to be independent and grown up is maybe not the sensible, modern way of living that people think it is. It is a strange way of keeping love and connection in our lives.

And the small things. What we offer and do. Again, these do not need to be remarkable. I am beginning to realise this. I have written Wendy so many love letters, these grand statements, but she would much prefer that I just talked with her, she would much prefer that I could play more naturally with the children than spend my time shopping and organising.

I said I do not do much for Mum and Dad when I am down with them, just the putting up and down of the sunshade in the garden, but that is the ritual: Graham puts up the sunshade in the morning, puts out the cushions and we sit and read in the garden, occasionally saying some brief words. It suits us, I think. We are not an excitable or voluble family and though, when I was with Wendy and her dad, there was a constant noise from the telly, the children, and her and her dad chattering, I do not think that it matters so much that we are different.

I think, however, we can wish that it had been different. Mum is like Wendy in that she is, by nature, sociable: always meeting up with friends, always nattering and laughing with them, so maybe there is something slightly sad at the silent evenings they now often have together but maybe not, maybe that very ability to be companionable is the really special thing.

2019—JUNE—MY MENTAL HEALTH AND ME— EXPLAINING THE PAST.

We went to the Cardross Inn with Peter and Sharon, Sophie and Lewis. It is lovely to be seeing so much of Wendy's brother's family. It is always a bit chaotic. With all of us combined, there are eight of us and Sharon is almost as enthusiastic about family and life as Wendy is. When Clare's family are with us too, it is thirteen of us.

We caused some nuisance by getting two outside tables lined up against each other so that they could fit all of us in one place. I was down where Charlotte and James were, and as usual, was looking after Dash who was being his lovely self. As it was a hot day, I had my shirt sleeves rolled up and as always happens, Sophie and Lewis, who both adore Dash, came to play with him and try to feed him chips and to stroke and pet him. Eventually, Charlotte squeezed up so that Sophie could sit beside her and Dash (and me). Sophie glanced at my arms and asked what all the scars were.

I don't remember how I replied. I think I was evasive, or knowing me, just didn't reply. She asked a couple more times, intrigued and confused by them. She is only a year older than Charlotte but physically she seems so much older, well into her teenage years. It must be hard for her, still being very young but maybe seen as more of an adult than she actually is. I still didn't tell her what the scars were. I thought I needed to check with her mum that she would be happy for me to let her know.

I suppose that is stigma: the keeping of self-harm secret from our children and the needing to ask permission of their parents if they ask about it. But maybe it is a prejudice against our children? A desire to keep them safe from a world that is not remotely safe? I don't know. I felt awkward and very uneasy. I do not like to keep secrets. But I do not like to distress young people with information that they do not understand or necessarily want to know about.

I am not necessarily ashamed but there seems to be something naff about saying, "Sometimes life is so bad for me that I want to slice chunks out of me. Sometimes life is so bad, I do not want to live. And that feeling carries on for day after day after day."

How do you reply to that in company if you are an adult? And how on earth would you reply to it if you are a child, like Charlotte, still snuggling into teddy bears and writing letters to fairies?

I texted Sharon later and said I would be happy for her to tell Sophie if she wanted and that led to a conversation with Wendy.

In the end it was, I think, a non event! We didn't mention the still want to die bit, but both Sophie and Charlotte, when speaking to their mothers, took it in their stride, were neither horrified nor disgusted. To be honest, I think that Charlotte, despite her youth, is even more tender with me than before she knew. James, as far as I know, was not interested at all!

July

2021—JULY—WENDY—BEING A DANDELION PARACHUTE AGAIN

I am whirling in the sunshine.

There I was, in one of our July thunderstorms, with the wind and the lightning and my sodden flapping clothes, being tossed way, way above the limits of breath and the land. It was difficult, to say the least. Far above the ground, streaming with water and loud angry birds. Hiding from the maelstrom, way above the drains, forced open by the pressure of the flood for dirty water to soak my shoes. I find I am flung this way and that, my mouth full of the sulphur taste of spent electrical explosions, my skin goosebump-covered, my muscles trembling uncontrollably, sending pain down my legs into my stomach and I am so lonely, so terribly lonely. This is where I live, clouded by memories I both strive to forget and strive uncertainly to believe were real. This is where I live, trying to work out how to find the lightness I am sure was once a part of me. Here I am, whirling, and I see my family shaking their heads, I see the tenderness of Wendy and the children, tired, crying a little.

I see the tenderness; I see the tenderness! I find I am a feather bathed by the sunshine, drifting down to earth; drying out, becoming light. I can smell the honeysuckle, the dog roses. I can smell elder blossom and the rich mud of the bay. I can smell the dark green moisture of the sun-dazzled, dappled woods. Everywhere there are bees droning in the sunshine. Just beside the last of the flag iris, I can see orange-tipped butterflies. In the fields, the lambs are growing, needing the shade of the trees at the edge of the field so much that they ignore the dogs walking on the path beside them. The cattle lie soft in the bright green of their tree-crowded field next to the bright yellow of the buttercup one.

I land lightly on the ground, ready to be waved aloft again in the next gust of wind. Dash the dog sniffs at me in a puzzled fashion and the children look at his skittish uncertainty. He gets close, gives a big sniff. I stick to his moist nose. The children burst out laughing. Dash paws at his nose and brushes me free. I rise unsteadily in a tiny zephyr of wind and then lose the breeze, tumble down to fall in Wendy's hair. She laughs and plucks me out to hold me in the palm of her hand. All uncertain, I lie there flickering slightly, about to whirl away again in the sunshine.

"Isn't it pretty!" she tells the children. "Who is going to carry it home? We can place it among the seaglass and the driftwood and make the house look nice."

"Oh, thank you." I whisper. "I never knew I was pretty. Can I stay here with you all for ever and ever?"

2021—JULY—MY JOURNAL

We are in the run up, we have passed midsummer. Each day will be shorter now and sometime, towards the very end of this book, we will reach the shortest day of the year. In contrast to the long days at present and the ever-present scent of flowers and blossom, the trees will be bare and the vegetation scarce.

It is a moment to take stock. I want you to reach the end of this book and hopefully leave, moved a little. I would love it if you could smile a little too and close the book tenderly, shut down the Kindle wistfully, maybe even wonder what I might write next.

On the first of this month, Wendy and I had a conversation, one of those important ones where you carry out some sort of reckoning. We reached some conclusions that are leading me to some further thoughts about what I want to give you with these words.

It is a decade since the children were born. Wendy is stretching her arms, saying, after a decade of concentrating almost exclusively on her children, and if not on them, on her dad or her mum or me, she needs to find some room for herself.

I wholeheartedly agree! If we go to a charity shop, she will look for things for the children; the Amazon parcels that come through the door are child-based. We work our week around the children. Wendy doesn't go out unless she is completely sure the children will be ok. When I go to bed, Wendy stays up late to get time for herself, going to sleep in the early hours and waking up tired. She is cross that she eats to give slight gifts of comfort to herself; cross that she is slightly overweight and does not feel good about it. She misses those years when she was always going out to dance or exercise or see friends and now she is saying maybe it is time for her to do something for herself and for us to help that happen. And of course it is! She is off just now for a weekend in Edinburgh with Sharon and Clare; it sounds wonderful but heavy rain and thunderstorms are forecast. I told her to take an umbrella and pack more clothes but she says she will be mainly inside, that there is no need to worry about such things.

I think my constant risk assessment adds to her frustration; my need to plan dinner every day; to keep the house full of food and drink, to know what we will be doing next week or in the evening.

It frustrates me hugely too. Just as Wendy wants to make changes for herself, so would I for myself. I said at the beginning of this book that the last five years have been a bit shit and they have. The weight of all of the things that have happened, some that I won't tell you about, hang heavy on me. I have become stolid and silent; I do not shine. I am weary.

When Wendy says she wants to get healthy, I agree but get cross when she says I could too. I could and I should but I like my whisky. I like eating too much and sleeping. I do not have the zest in me to take a hold of my life. I really do have the most perfect of lives, but the chance of us getting chucked out of a bus station again because we are kissing too intimately seems remote; our giggles that we might be seen from the path because we have found a glade to be naked in is so far away from our lives now. Who wants to be grabbed by a person with passion when he seeks certainty and permission for every little thing, makes lists for how to live? Who doubts his lover's love and his family's love, even though all the evidence demonstrates it again and again, and asks over and over for reassurance about it? Who trembles with excitement at a partner who cannot talk in company? Never has a clue about what to do unless it is to take Dash the dog for a walk or to put the bins out on a Sunday?

Instead, I remember this time last year when Sandy told me his cancer was now in his liver and that I would need to help Wendy. At the time I was in Dublin, speaking at a conference, but my attempts at support and sympathy were so crass that Wendy had to put the phone down in tears.

I miss those years when it was simpler and Wendy knew me, in Nairn, when I had so many friends, when each time she visited she had to carve space for us because there were so many people I wanted her to see, so many things I wanted to do.

I really know no one down here and do not know how to get to know people or even how to speak to them. Wendy is my main company. I would not go out for coffee or lunch with another person unless it was a work thing. I would not set off camping with Dash, even though I would love to. I would not take us all away to an island, or anywhere really.

From being the person who initiated a lot of things, I am now the person who asks for help. The laptops and the internet? When those things go wrong, I panic, turn to Wendy. Ordering online? Wendy has Amazon Prime. Get work done on the house? Wendy knows the best ways to find people. It is so easy to see why Wendy would love chances to be free of responsibility, just to laugh and enjoy herself.

It is easy to see why, when Wendy asks me what I would like to change, I say that I would like to live a little, to find joy in my heart; have the energy to become the person who doesn't make lists, the person who couldn't care less if we run out of bread or toilet roll! The person who is confident enough to tease James until he is weak with giggles. The person who can ask Charlotte something other than how school was or what she would like for breakfast.

When I said that, I remember that Wendy laughed at my ambition; wondered how I could change who I am; asked how I could get beyond the illness bits that she thinks make me like this? And at the same time said, yes of course we must try to find ways out of the bonds we have constructed around ourselves.

And we can! I just mentioned that Wendy is in Edinburgh this weekend, busy partying! A couple of days ago I was taking the children fruit picking near Glasgow airport and they were laughing so much, when not long before we doubted they would agree to go there alone with me. A day ago I went to creative writing at Jean's Bothy and, for the first time in two years there, managed to witter and laugh. I repeated it again today at the photography. These are signs that change is possible.

I think the weight of the years have served to make me divide the day into manageable chunks; to order everything. I write my book. This book! But somehow I discarded my sense of humour, my sense of fun. I lost my delight in finding that life could be free and full of dandelion blossom. My belief that everything was wonderful took a nosedive and it is no wonder. People dying, lockdown, illness, stressful jobs, carved the light right away from me.

I want to find it again and I want to find out what I really feel about my dad. I find it very strange that I got so angry with my dad when I didn't find the affection and love I had wanted to find in his memoir. I had thought that all the recent years that I keep coming across in the Facebook Memories with my dad, had removed the last vestiges of the resentment I carried. I thought that last tear-stained loving declaration that we loved each other was such a gift of a parting that it made his death something that was possible to live beyond, relatively painlessly, but I find I wanted something else and, much as I peer around me, I am not sure what it was.

I find I can write a whole book which has as much of its core, my dad, when really my contact with him was limited. He was a big man, an angry man, a vibrant man and latterly, a gentle and loving man. I know full well people of his generation did not expect to be fathers in the way we are expected to be now and did not express emotion in the way we are expected to now, so why do I feel an absence and a resentment? Why can't I just remember with joy all those days in his garden and trips to the seafront with him in his buggy or special treats of lunch in restaurants? Why do I write this all down?

I speak to my mum every day; we tease each other and giggle; she often tells me I am lazy and I often tell her she is too busy. I could not write a book about her. I could not even summarise our daily conversations, they just are! I take them for granted. I have no need at all to write them down: Mum is Mum. I love her, she loves me, what more do I need to say? Why would I not write a book about her? Why don't I know what I would put in it? The conversations we have, despite seeming inconsequential, are the very essence of all that is important in life.

She is a much better person than my dad and I combined and yet I constantly strive in this writing to understand my dad. I know he ended up very proud of me, I know he envied me some of my good fortune. I think, though I grasp for straws here, I think I wish that many years ago, way before I don't know what, that I had known I was loved and that I was valued. My memory is so faulty here, but I would like it if he had played with me, read me books in the evening, not sent me away, that sort of thing.

I think maybe where I want to be by the end of the book is to gain the feeling that my sister has that Dad just slipped away. Something gentle and unremarkable. I want to realise that making sense of things like this

Edinburgh's Radical Book Fair

9 - 12th
November 2023

Hosted by the
Lighthouse Bookshop
at Assembly Roxy
in Edinburgh's Old Town

Details & Tickets:
www.lighthousebookshop.com

Revolutionary Feeling

RADICAL BOOK FAIR

NOV 2023
09-12

STALLS + WORKSHOPS + EVENTS

THURSDAY 9TH

Book Fair free to browse 12pm-7pm

Gary Younge: from Nelson Mandela to Black Lives Matter 5.30pm

The Stories We Bring: Suhaiymah Manzoor-Khan / Matt Colquhoun / Nathalie Olah 7.30pm

---

FRIDAY 10TH

Book Fair free to browse 10am-7pm

Lavender Menace x Kate Charlesworth 12.00pm

A Picture is Worth a Thousand Words: Creative Workshop with Celeste John Wood 12.15pm

Abolition Here & Everywhere: Phil Crockett Thomas / Glasgow Prisoner Solidarity / JJ Fakada 1.30pm

Read Think Act: Yara Rodrigues Fowler / Left Cultures / Yasmin El-Rifae 5.30pm

This Thread of Gold: A night of Performance ft. Catherine Joy White / Gemma Cairney 7.30pm

---

SATURDAY 11TH

Book Fair free to browse 10am-7pm

Blunt Knife Zine Workshop 10.00am

No Platform: Solidarity & Censorship from BDS to Trans rights 11.00am

New Intimacies: Hannah Silva / Lynne Segal / Sophie Chauhan 12.30pm

Climate Power shifts: Quan Nguyen / James Marriott / Terry Macalister 2.30pm

A World to Live For: Charlie Hertzog-Young / Nadia Karim / Jessica Gaitán Johannesson 4.30pm

Alliances in the Making: Arianne Shahvisi / Jenni Keasden / Mohamed Tonsy 6.00pm

Feminist Cabaret: Titi Farukuoye / Lisa Fannen / Lakshmi Ajay / Aliya Davids 8.00pm

---

SUNDAY 12TH

Book Fair free to browse 10am-6pm

Pandemics of Inequality: Nick Dearden / Saleyha Ahsan / Leah Hazard 11.00am

Free to Decide: reproductive rights for all ft. Kirsty Logan / Sian Norris / Alice Spawls 12.30pm

Adapt or Remake: Micha Frazer Carroll / Robert Chapman / Fiona Robertson 2.30pm

Right to the Center: Online extremism and how to resist ft. Alice Capelle 4.30pm

Neil Davidson Lecture: Raquel Varela 6.30pm

TICKETS + INFO
LIGHTHOUSEBOOKSHOP.COM

ASSEMBLY ROXY
2 ROXBURGH PL, EDINBURGH EH8 9SU

is really pretty unnecessary. Rather than studying my life, I hope that by the time I reach 2022, I have found it within me to restart the living stuff. Rather than Wendy coming home tomorrow, looking forward to my gentleness, my quietness, that reassuring background love, I want her to be excited to see me again, like she was a few years ago before life swiped us sideways. I want, sometime around Christmas, to find somewhere, the laughter and energy I am sure I once had, and I want to stop thinking that this heavy soul, this blunt-shadowed version of me is a sign of this schizophrenia stuff.

I want to reject that all over again. Even if it is true, I want to reject it because if that is how my life will be for the next few decades then it will be unbearable and those I love so much will suffer even more than they do now, with me presently inhabiting this screen in which I hide.

That feels good! I am going to search for humour. I am going to search for the hope that my quixotic rejection of my illness gives me. I will learn, step by painful step, how to live again and hopefully, by the time I realise I have been doing it all along, I will no longer need to remind myself of such simple lessons.

2021—JULY—ALAN—MORE AND MORE, I COMPARE US.

I find myself perplexed and afraid I am being harder than I have any need to be on my dad. My dad's career? I have just read a whole memoir about it.

Maybe I should be more conscious of his career. I imagine he is mentioned here and there in some papers about the RAF and Lightnings and Phantoms and Typhoons and that there are bound to be records of his service and the squadrons he flew in. I know when I was very young I was very impressed by his job, especially by his uniform. However,

I mainly remember walks with the dog and the rest of the family. I remember being sure that having a fighter pilot as a dad was far better than having a potter for a dad and all the other different jobs we knew our dads did.

And his yachts. I was about to say I mainly remember him shouting at us when we got one of his high speed berthing exercises wrong in front of the public, or when we got the spinnaker wrong when taking prospective buyers for a sail. Or maybe the many times we had to clear up the mess after clients were seasick. Or those long, long nights of being polite waiters when entertaining clients at the dinner table at home. Or the boat shows, passing out fliers, learning how to take visitors round the boat. Or day after day of deck scrubbing, hull polishing, winch maintenance, rope whipping and splicing. But I think that is cruel. Family businesses are like that. You get involved young, whether you like it or not.

His dream was for one of us to take over his business, to make it flourish. He did all he could with Richard and I, less so with Juliet, to make sure we knew the business and techniques of sailing. Our summer holidays always involved whatever the latest demonstrator boat was and I have to admit that wasn't bad. When he wasn't shouting and telling us what to do, we went on some wonderful trips. Over to the Channel Islands and to France and later, sailing on much posher yachts where we had freezers and air conditioning, in the Mediterranean; stopping at islands to have lamb roasted over rosemary fires and to drink wine.

Those nights sailing between islands were lovely, seeing Stromboli erupting as we drifted past, putting into small anchorages on our way to deliver a yacht to Dubrovnik. Those were times when his business really fell into family life and could be truly wonderful.

Even some of the more unpleasant delivery trips were sometimes special. I will never forget sailing through a gale in the driving rain and in the path of migrating birds and how I was at the helm, stood with my legs splayed for balance in the cockpit and a songbird flew into the cockpit and crawled up my leg until it was sheltered from the rain by my oilskins and how I needed to make sure I did not disturb it until it was dry and ready to continue its journey.

Or the time on the Irish Sea when all the crew and the new owner were drunk and most were seasick; we had been sailing in gales for a week, seeing water spouts, plunging ferries. Or when he praised Richard and I for a very difficult course change when we were a bit too young for crewing and Dad had realised the weather was far too bad for us to get to the boat show and that we needed to go back the way we came.

Yes. There really were some wonderful times. I became a good sailor ultimately, but not that good. I could do it; I could just about skipper a yacht, do the navigation, manage the watches and sleeplessness, cope with gales and broken things, but I am not a natural. I do not like taking risks and I do not think quickly and logically, and I am not practical. My dad said he would rather sail with me in a gale than anyone else, but I am not at all sure about that anymore. I think that was my dad's way of being a dad. His version of kindness.

His ambition was immense, and he was always on the verge of tremendous success. And those yachts really were beautiful; they gave joy, even to the onlookers who watched them sail past.

But is it what he really wanted? I have no idea. I know much of his working life was difficult. It meant mixing with millionaires routinely, which I think he liked, but it also meant pacifying them just because they wanted to be pacified. It meant employing people but I fear his standards and temper did not make for a good combination. We got terrible rows from Dad and sometimes gained comfort from workers saying he should never have spoken to us like that, but he also employed and sacked people with a frequency that should maybe have made him consider his judgement.

Of course, it also meant huge financial uncertainty, with everything on the line for whatever his latest venture was. He worked incredibly hard, was endlessly creative; my mum worked terribly hard and incredibly efficiently alongside him. I really don't know if it is what he wanted. I remember recently, Mum saying he did all the things he loved in his life: the sailing, the flying, the sea, adventure; that he had the life he set out to have. That sounds so good and makes me wonder why I am uncertain.

We joined in, I suppose. The weeks of doing the accounts and the receipts over a summer's holiday do not rest well with me. Being beholden and loyal both to him and the new owner of a yacht in Taiwan was an impossibility that did not end well.

And my whatever it was.

Were my years of silence and resentment and anger and confusion the prodromal signs of schizophrenia? Some people say they were. Maybe if I had known, and had ever believed that, might life with my dad have been very different? Instead of what I sometimes still feel when I am maudlin, a justified resentment of his manipulation, anger and controlling ways, might we have worked together, seen the same sunsets, surfed massive yachts down waves? Might I have learnt the complexities of sailing and design and business that could have made for a very different life?

However, I knew very early on that I would not survive in his business and did not want to join it, and that if I had it would probably have been a disaster. If I had been different, or if my dad had been different, maybe we would have had a very different life. Maybe I would have spent most of my life sailing, commissioning and selling incredible yachts to very, very rich people and that might have been amazing. There is, after all, so much wonder and beauty at sea.

I might have ended up so much more financially secure than I have ever been and my dad might have retired thinking he had made a success of his business rather than ultimately selling it for £1 and, in the last few years, apologising for what he felt he did to me and for his own messed up emotional landscape.

I think it is sad and find it hard to recognise that I fell into much the same trap.

In order to feel value and worth I went down a very different line of justice and rights, and in the extremely niche and small world I inhabit, I have been extremely successful at it in much the same, not quite successful way of my dad. But that is a slightly silly way of looking at it and when I look at friends and family and what they have made of their lives, very silly indeed.

I focussed so earnestly on work, worked till I cracked up, worked till I could hardly speak when I was home, worked so I didn't get home till after my son was in bed. I worked to validate myself so much that I was exhausted and had neither the time or realisation that my family could have benefited from my company; scant chance of interaction when I could do little more than lift a whisky glass to my lips when I got home.

I still work hard. I am working now, if this could be called work, at the end of my holidays. I am really, really hoping that when Wendy gets home from celebrating her mum's birthday that I do whatever it might be that allows her to relax and feel loved and looked after in the way I doubt my ex-wife ever felt.

I really hope my last five days of holiday have, at least on occasion, helped the children feel some joy in my company as well as their mum's.

I really hope in the clichéd trope that I have recently learnt that when I reach the end of my life it really won't be whether I have helped fashion forward-looking legislation or helped promote our rights and awareness. I hope it is that for however long it is, that Dash will sleep with his head on my feet as he is now; that Charlotte will continue to cuddle me and say, "Goodbye, I love you!" when going off to her dad's and James will continue to giggle at his new nickname for me of 'Rock face'!

2021—JULY—MENTAL HEALTH AND ME— LOCKDOWN AND MY MENTAL HEALTH TEAM

I need to introduce you to Mairi. She was my CPN until just before lockdown. A lovely woman, young, pretty, she has two children, a partner and was just good at being human. It took me ages and ages to trust her and by that I mean, years. I am not sure what she did that made me trust her. I think it was as simple as the fact that she said she liked coming to visit us and that she always had words for Wendy and the children and liked the dog. We did not talk much about illness or anything like that; more often we nattered about holidays in Amsterdam or spa days. But I felt that she kept an eye on me and knew when I was struggling. She made me feel safe.

And feeling safe is a precious feeling.

Lockdown came not long after Mairi left for a different job. I didn't really have a permanent CPN after Mairi left. I would turn up every two weeks for my jag and someone or other would give me my jag and I would leave.

When the announcement of lockdown came, I had a talk with a CPN who did not quite know what to do. He started off saying they might not be able to see me and that I might have to take medication willingly instead of getting a jag; then that scheme got shelved and he said he really was not at all sure what would happen if I got any symptoms and still needed my jag.

Not long after that, the mental health team shut up shop and moved across to Dumbarton. It felt a bit weird really, almost as though all help had stopped.

It didn't worry me too much, to be honest. I was loving lockdown. It meant I no longer had to travel across the country to work. It meant I could get up later and take breaks to take the children and Dash the dog out for wanders with Wendy. The weather was good. I hadn't lost my job and it didn't seem like I would, and neither had Wendy. I created my office in the bedroom and worked away.

Every two weeks, I would go for my jag. Off to the Joint Hospital with my mask and my hands smeared with gel. Trying to ring the bell to the clinic with my elbow, mindful of the notice on the door saying that they weren't seeing clients except by appointment. If all my treatment consisted of was getting some drugs into my body, the arrangement was very effective; if it should also have involved saying how I was feeling or coping, or if I had any problems, it was useless.

I just do not speak to complete strangers about how I am coping or feeling, and complete strangers in all their PPE at the opposite end of the room, trying to spend as little an amount of time in my company as they could manage, didn't help. I don't even remember any of the names of all the different people who came out of their office to jag me. I am sure some were nice and some not so nice, maybe they were all nice but I am not entirely sure.

I was lucky by the time life fell apart again that I had a new CPN and was going back to the newly re-established mental health team in Helensburgh and my new CPN, if my memory is correct, is the one I still have. She is good, I think. I am much more alert and funny with her than I am in real life. I don't think she sees me as anything other than a patient, that the boundaries of being a professional are well and truly in place but I tend to find I can talk to her.

I've seen my psychiatrist once since lockdown, that time he renewed my CTO. I had a go at speaking to him on the phone but that didn't go so well and I am meant to be speaking to him on the phone again soon. He did write me a very helpful letter when my PIP review happened which I hope will help with their decision about my future.

I wanted to go to Jean's Bothy which is a wellbeing hub that I love but am shy about. They put everything online, had chill and chats and yoga and writing and all sorts of things. For some reason, although I was running my own Zoom meetings for work, when I joined Zoom meetings for Jean's Bothy, I felt unable to join in. I just couldn't. They encouraged me and it was welcoming but I remained silent. I kept myself muted and then kept my camera off and then I avoided going along altogether.

That is until some time this year, just as lockdown was diminishing. I joined the photography group and kept popping by to pick up food that they had for people. It was out of date food and would have gone to the bin if we didn't get it, so it felt good to use it. I started writing for the newsletter, joined the book group. Finally I feel confident about walking into the garden and feel that I can smile at people when I go there, maybe even talk or make a joke. It feels wonderful.

I don't know why it feels wonderful but I feel I belong and am accepted; that if I need help I can go there. I feel that I am welcome and valued.

The very best bit was just before Christmas last year, just as I was beginning to get involved with them more actively. We got back from a day out and found an unexpected parcel on the doorstep. It was full of chocolate and coffee and different goodies. For some reason it took my breath away, it just seemed so kind that I, more or less a stranger, would be given an unexpected present for me and the family by the drop-in I was still a bit uncertain about. I felt so treasured and valued; for some reason that made me feel like crying.

I don't know if my mental health has suffered because of lockdown. I am less sociable than many, less able to pick up on cues of behaviour and emotion. I find people difficult and tiring but at the same time I love to be with them. I miss being with people on a ferry to Mull, or wandering off to buy Arbroath Smokies after another meeting there. But I like that I am home most of the time, with my family, with the dog but seeing people you know so well on the screen; somehow you are interacting but at the same time are not, that is confusing.

I am unsure of my mental health team; they jag me, ask me some questions, see how I have been getting on; say they are always there if I need them. There have been times these last two years when I would have wanted something. I want to come to terms with that teacher, and I want to come to terms with whatever the reality of some of my childhood was and I would like to come to terms with the horror my marriage became and the fact that I will probably never see my son again. Somehow those things are not options and when they are, they quickly backtrack and say addressing such things at this time could be too risky to my wellbeing and then I retreat. I stop talking about being lost from myself, stop saying anything much at all. I still say thank you when they have given me the jag I don't want to take. It seems polite, maybe a courtesy to those trying to help me.

August

2021—AUGUST—WENDY—THE CERTAINTY OF HOME THAT BRIGHTENS MY SOUL

I tend to go to bed around nine thirty or ten in the evening. I like the moments of peace that I get before I fall asleep. I like the chance to feel the smoothness of my bed, the feel of Dash resting his head on my feet, to feel the coolness of the wind on my chest because I have left the window open.

At this time of year, the night is just beginning when I take Dash out for his last wee. The sun will have just set and the sky will have the remnants of the sunset in it, or the tinges of the blueness that heralds the black of the night.

I love these moments. Dash sniffs all along the path and into the woods beside the pavement. Sometimes he uncovers a hedgehog; always we will hear the rooks settling down, way above us in the trees, almost as though they have returned all excited and slightly argumentative after a night out at the pub. The stragglers will still be swooping down from the last light of the sky. As we walk along there is also always a clattering of something falling from the trees. I have feeling that they don't like Dash and I walking below them, or nearly below them, and that they are busy pooing away their displeasure but really, I have no idea.

As we walk along and our eyes adjust, we see tiny shapes flittering about us, totally silent and flittering, not fluttering. They are quick and purposeful and switch direction all the time. If I look up and see them outlined against the sky, I can see that they are tiny bats. I love it, I really love it. They fill me with an awe and some sort of excitement that I cannot quite name.

When we turn around to go back to the house, if the curtains are not closed, which is usually the case, I will see the big driftwood love heart that I gave Wendy one Christmas, attached to the wall, with the light of the room spilling out into the street. When I walk up to the house, I tend to get dunted by the clump of roses that hang above the door and once I walk into the house, you will call out from the sofa, "How did you two get on?" which I always find strange because we go out for Dash's wee every evening and it is almost always much the same. But I like that you ask.

Before I go up to the bedroom with Dash, we will share a good night kiss. If we were less tired we would share much more than a kiss and sometimes we do, but that touch of your lips and your smile when we break apart makes me shine happily.

Walking is not really your thing, especially doing the same walk again and again and again. Nowadays, when I walk at Ardmore I can see the season is turning. There are still flowers out, the daisies still flutter in the wind, the ragwort still bobs on the sea wall, the rosebay willow herbs still look lovely. The Himalayan balsam is just beginning to flourish and overpower the paths with its scent, but on the path I am beginning to see the yellow patches of fallen birch leaves, the multi-coloured shells of sycamore leaves, the dog roses are still out but there are also swollen rose hips on the same stem. The rowan berries are beginning to ripen; the brambles are showing patches of plump darkness among their hard red sisters.

I love it. The wind is still warm and I still don't really need wellies or coats or jumpers to walk the path, but at the edge of my mind, I can see the dark mornings: Dash refusing to get out the car, me trying to get my boots on without getting my socks wet, the wind burning my skin with its coldness.

But for the moment, I will remember that just like today, you will be at home, ready to call out again, "How did you two get on?" as I place my keys on their hook, my bag where the coats hang, the lead on the old wooden bench, while Dash rushes into the sitting room to lick a welcome on you while he waits for his dinner to appear in his bowl.

Well, for the moment, summer is over. This morning I saw pictures of cars submerged in floods in the Vale, across the hill from us, and just now got soaked when I had to run to and from the car so that Dot and her children could get home relatively dry. Still, the pond will be full, the flowers will be watered.

I have spent some evenings with Wendy, watching films recently, all snuggled up; a lovely feeling. One of the films we watched was *My Big Fat Greek Wedding*. At the end Wendy said that the father reminded her of my dad in a really nice way. And he does, now I think of it, an outrageous patriarch, who dominates and bullies the family but under his bluster and passion is someone totally in love with his family, capable of great generosity.

I can see that in my dad. I remember in his later years when he was so good at giving hugs and saying he loved us. I like this vision much more than the one that has been consuming me over the past few weeks. I like the idea of finding out that I did really love my dad just as I thought I did.

It is strange how we can create stories about the people in our lives, that our perspective can shift and grow and that this is maybe as much a product of what we want and need as the reality of those around us. It makes me feel more tender and less angry and less upset. He has even appeared in my dreams again, which is a welcome return. As usual, I find myself sailing up weird Mediterranean estuaries on very posh yachts. It is a little like having a holiday in your sleep.

Last night's sleep was one of my bad ones; not as bad in terms of sleep as in the past, but a confused series of nightmares that I became aware of at around four a.m. I am no longer quite clear what they were but I know they involved people with extreme beliefs who did not approve of me. I remember that I dreamt I had told Wendy about my nightmares and that some hours later was still involved in them, wandering down some strange and frightening street, with a series of inadequate possessions strung over my shoulder, being deliberately not told where I needed so desperately to go.

My policeman has now sent me my statement about the school for approval which is a slightly strange feeling. I am meant to be getting people who remember me talking about it in the past to confirm that they heard me say such things. Apparently, it gives greater credibility to what I say, but so far no one remembers apart from Wendy, which is a bit frustrating.

This month has been one where we have been busy at work and busy trying to give the children bits of joy within their holidays while we work away in between. For the first time in a very long time I am happy in my work. However, I am very aware now that I am deeply suspicious of people. In the Scott Review, I am sure some of the executive despise me and even more people from the secretariat. But no one has said anything approaching that. To be honest, two people from the secretariat have been open in their admiration of what I have been doing. This pleases me so much, but at the same time I worry that they have been instructed to make me feel good because I am so adept at feeling bad about the review.

At work I worry that a report I finished six months ago is not going to be completed because it seems no nearer being published than when I passed it on all those months ago. But again, I have no evidence that there is any intent to that, I think because it isn't true.

I panicked when I did my writing workshop for the arts festival, especially as the other workshops were run by writers who are so famous that even I have heard of them, but somehow it all worked out fine. I am seeing a journalist next week but am not entirely sure why; his wife is also a writer and has read my book, but I worry that they will hate me when they actually meet me. But for the first time in a long time I am not too bothered by how much most people despise me and look down on me. Instead, I do my meetings, write my speeches, hold discussions and feel that I do a fairly good job of what I do, and that if I don't I will not worry too much about it.

So much of my life is a maze of worry and suspicion. It can be exhausting when I prepare for meetings and assume that people will have heard of me before and will be waiting for me unwillingly, oozing contempt. And yet it is so incredibly rare that people are unkind to me; most people are lovely; most people accommodate my silence and awkwardness, overlook my embarrassingly palpable need to be loved and admired.

Wendy says I have all the elements of a newly-listed disorder called Boarding School Syndrome and, though I laugh about it, I know that I do, but enough of that! Let's get back to the holidays.

We went to M&D's and scooted around on the dodgems, the elephant ride, the caterpillar train. We ate freshly fried doughnuts and sat on the grass with Dash the dog peering all around him. We went to the cinema to see *The Croods* and all of us giggled, felt happy as we left. We went to Culzean Castle minus James, slightly unaware just how far away it was from home. By the time we were finally parked, I was tight-lipped about something or other but as soon as Dash and I walked by the swan pond with its lilies and willow sculptures, I felt my heart relax with the joy of it. Charlotte played in the adventure park; we ate ice creams and sausage rolls, vegan sausage rolls in my case. We walked in the woods above the high cliffs. We wandered round the edge of the castle. Wendy said that she would have had the most idyllic life if she had been brought up as a child of the lord, or whoever he was, and that this is what her life should have been! Charlotte got a sore leg. We sat on the beach by the marram grass and watched the waves. It was so lovely.

Today I went to my photography course at Jean's Bothy and basked in my ability to relax there. We teased each other and pretended I know what I am talking about when I so definitely don't. Kath patiently teaches us and I think we all feel slightly awed that our pictures will be used for an exhibition and maybe end up in a calendar or book.

Now I have an afternoon free to myself. Wendy is in Dumbarton with her mum to visit the charity shops and drink coffee. She tells me she will make her own way home as long as her endometriosis does not get too bad.

It is like this every month. It is like a *Truman Show* thing. She is always so surprised at how tired she gets, at how much pain she is in and how slowly and foggily her brain works, and I always irritate her by saying, this time we must phone the doctor for an appointment. She always agrees she will but as soon as the pain ebbs away, she puts it behind her and forgets until it inevitably returns, this time just a bit more ruthless in its pain than before.

I am even more surprised at how lucky I am with my life nowadays. Each adventure we have originates from Wendy, each celebration comes from her. If there are peals of laughter from the children they will have originated from something she has done. If the children are down and low, she will cuddle up to them and talk to them until they feel more confident. If I am being pompous or arrogant, she will make me giggle at my silliness. If I am being silent, she will tell me to remember to use my words and we will both laugh.

I do not really know what I bring to this house and yet, yesterday, when Charlotte was talking about her feelings about her mummy and daddy splitting up, she said, "But if you hadn't done that, I would never have met Graham, so it was good that you did."

That delights me and totally bemuses me. I don't do much more than walk the dog, do the washing, shopping and cooking and occasionally grunt at people!

The children are off to school again on Monday. That will be strange.

I have got used to long lies and fitting work around play and outings. I have enjoyed it very much.

An addendum: last week, I went to Edinburgh to do my first work away from home in ages. On the way, I found out that my lovely, lovely, charming niece, Keri, who has so recently struggled through rehab, struggled through homelessness, had jumped off a Glasgow bridge. She has now had three operations on her shattered legs, is in agony and needs a skin graft for where one of her legs was sliced open when she got compartment syndrome. It breaks my heart a little. She is such a wonderful person and in so much pain. If I can, I will write about her more. I left her out in earlier months because I was not sure she would like to be mentioned but now in my tale of this year, I am not sure I can any more.

It seems so long ago, but it was only three years ago that we went to visit Sandy who had been under the weather for a few days. It is a vivid but also distant memory that when we arrived we found out that he was extremely ill: ambulances to hospital, a busy Accident and Emergency, us not understanding why we were in the relatives resus room until a doctor explained that Sandy was unlikely to survive the night. Then days and days of trips to the hospital; no time to cook, work when possible, pick the children up from school; off to Morrison's café, which we began to hate, off to the hospital, to a single room because of infection control. Drips and oxygen masks. Charlotte perched on my knee, James on Wendy's. Wendy telling tales of our day and the highlights of the dramas of our lives. Sandy at his very, very worst on some days, just staring silently at the ceiling. Charlotte whispering to me that she knew he was dying but was he 100% dying? James insisting he wasn't dying. Then finally to the discovery that he also had bowel cancer and the decision to operate. Not to cure but to avoid a very quick and painful death.

Those hours of waiting and Wendy's unbearable guilt when they phoned to say he would probably live but the next few hours would be critical; her wild tears because she didn't want him to carry on suffering and yet wanted her dad to live too; her trying to make sure the children didn't see how desperately upset she was so that they didn't, in turn, crumble.

That was when we promised ourselves we would visit him every day from then on and give him all we could to make his last months as good as they could be. They were also the start of almost the greatest tiredness either of us have ever experienced because, as I said at the beginning, all the other bits of life carried on: walking the dog, making meals, entertaining and looking after the children, school, work…

2021—AUGUST—ALAN—ALL AT SEA WITH MY DAD

My main memories, now I look back, the ones that resonate and I want to talk about, are about sailing with my dad. I have others which are harsher and less kind but I feel little need to mention them. As someone might say, they do not add to the story, might even be gratuitous.

As much as I peer into the last 58 years, I cannot see my dad in a form that I am confident of repeating. I know he loved discussion or – as I called it – argument, at the dining table. I know he felt that he had the right to be in charge and decide what we did and when we did it. That he sat at the head of the table and expected things to be done for him. But there really was that generous, loving side to him and those ticks of almost adorable uncertainty when you could see his face rehearsing what to say next.

Though I know my mum regretted it, and so did my dad, I welcomed his mellowing as he got older and went through treatment for cancer and had operations on his back. He seemed softer and kinder and more reflective, easier to be with.

When he and my mum took to taking their holidays with me after I left my wife, I found that I really looked forward to seeing them, that I no longer expected, at some point, an evening of bitter drunken recriminations, and no longer assumed we would have some loud and unnecessary discussion about politics or social issues. It was a relief to just enjoy time with them; to sit in the house waiting for my mum to come back from her morning walk on Nairn east beach, while Dad sat reading his paper by the window.

I think maybe the first memory of us really being at sea was down in Devon when we were very young. For a very short time, I think we owned some sort of dinghy. On a sunny day, we went out sailing. I remember a red hull, white sails, Richard and I with lifejackets on, being taught to trail lines for mackerel; that slight thrumming as we held our hands over the side and the tug as we pulled the line back and forward, to be replaced by the thrill and the fear when we got a much bigger tug and pulled the fish to the boat, its belly flashing in the sun as it got close to us. I do not remember how it came aboard or how it came off its hook, but I do remember that my dad smashed it violently over the head with something. So violently that the mainsail was speckled with bright red droplets of blood. My mum told me later that my dad was very squeamish about killing and gutting things. On the shore, my mum prepared the fish and cooked them, I remember being told that fish eaten fresh from the sea was the very best.

I remember being mid channel, the wind in our hair, the spray flicking back rapidly in an arc as the bows of the yacht went through the waves, the sunshine, sitting up on the far side of the cockpit. Anchorages where the sun goes down and you can hear the water lapping against the hull as we fall asleep while our parents talk in the cockpit.

That time we woke in the night to the sound of the yacht bumping on the rocks as my dad had got the anchorage or the tide wrong. Out in the dinghy with the boom wide across the water, trying to lever the boat sideways and free the keel until suddenly there was silence and smoothness as either the tide lifted us or we had edged ourselves off the rocks. Whatever it was that happened, we were free and motored out onto the Normandy coast with its rocks and islands and fast tides. I have glimpses in my mind of the night and the clouds and that sudden moment when we saw distress flares and had to take a bearing of them and my dad had to report the boat in distress to the coastguard. I also remember he told us what a good job we had done that night and can almost feel that warm, embarrassed, very awkward feeling of being complimented.

So many lunches at sea, watered down wine for us, baguettes, cheese, salami, fruit and salad and the wake of the boat behind us while Dad tried to teach us to steer with just the tips of our fingers, the slightest movement of the helm anticipating the waves and the wind and then those other times where everything is noise and movement and spray and flapping and the task of keeping a course is a major physical and rhythmical feat.

Or that time, off Land's End on our way to Bristol, where Richard, trying to fill a bucket with seawater for the washing, had it ripped out of his hands by the rush of the water and my dad decided this would be an ideal opportunity to practice man overboard drill. Round and round we went, coming up in the green sliced waves towards the bucket with our boathooks outstretched, only to eventually give up and leave it to its journey in the sea.

Better to remember are the times, late at night, when Dad was at the chart table, listening to the shipping forecast with the dim red glow of the night lights and the scratch of his pencil, or the smooth rush in the Med, under the stars where we talked in soft voices and drank chocolate or Cup a Soups at two in the morning. Or that time when we were setting off from Brighton in yet another gale and the owner was celebrating in a restaurant, and I had steak and kidney pudding. Maybe slipping through the water, us perched on the pulpit trying to dangle our legs in the water or lying on the foredeck in the sun or maybe off watch, listening to dolphins through the hull.

Or moored in a tiny bay at a tiny island, off Croatia, with wine in dumpy glasses, to finish with swimming in the bay or up further north in Krk, having a full bottle of chilled slivovitz placed on the table where we sat in a square with old buildings in the evening sun. That time near Dubrovnik where the forest fires nearly overran the marina and we were taken out of our beds to sit waiting while fire hoses snaked around our feet.

Or maybe, when we were slow to act, our dad with his strong arms winding fast on winches in ways we couldn't, or laughing with the joy of being at sea or sitting in a restaurant after we moored up for an evening.

My memory has tripped me up. I spent so many years being a victim of the misery of what I thought my upbringing was that I struggle to see what I know was mainly a wonderful time. I remember that tight, warm and tired skin after a day of sun and salt and wind, sitting down below, eating tea. I remember when the salt had semi-crystalised on the fibreglass; being taken to restaurants in the evening at the end of the day when all the boat show exhibitors had gathered for drinks to wind down, with the whole arena deserted.

I like that I can remember salt spray and sunny days, I like that I remember him carefully sipping the dash of wine in the bottom of a glass before letting the waiter pour the rest. I like the memory of the sheer physical strength of him, his vigour and dynamism, his deep, deep permanent brown tan.

There are other memories I am not sure need repeated or reported on and, despite my flinch, at what I have said is a bad memory, it is also one I really like: that he spent years getting drunk in order to tell me that he loved me and so that he could hug me and so that he could apologise to me.

I think I would like to relax enough to find glimpses of my life with him and to find out how good those could be. I would like to keep on seeing him in my dreams. I really like the person I see there and my feelings towards him. There is always a sense of family and doing things together or for him. I spent so many years denying family that finding it again and again when I sleep is wonderful.

2021—AUGUST—MENTAL HEALTH AND ME— WHEN LIFE WAS KINDER: REFLECTIONS OF A DISILLUSIONED MENTAL HEALTH ACTIVIST

Nearly forty years ago it all seemed so obvious. Newly released from one of the old asylums where I had stayed just long enough to be utterly scandalised by my treatment and that of my fellow patients, I embarked on a career of activism for the right for the voices of people like me, with a mental illness, to be heard, listened to and acted on.

I remember we thrilled at the halfway house, where we volunteered, and at the education of the radical workers who worked there. We really were like little disciples, drinking in, without question or reflection, the teachings of anti-psychiatry and critical psychiatry. For someone like me: young, anxious, distressed and filled with anger about what I still do not quite know, this seemed like an ideal cause to align myself to. Even more ideal, because as a white, middle class young man, I had so far had nothing to make me feel oppressed or exploited and I so needed a cause to engage in.

To describe our actions as misguided and naive would be very wrong. We did do some good things. I particularly enjoy the memory of setting up McMurphy's – a drop-in centre run by young people with a mental illness for young people with a mental illness, which we painfully created step by step and yet with such joy and excitement. Sometimes when I look back I wish that had been the path I had followed in my life; just creating the services and the culture we knew we thrived in, but I took a different path of activism and the expression of our voice.

It was very early in my career when I was still at university that I questioned my certainty and my anger at the professionals who had by then only featured briefly in my life. My parents, in a well-meaning attempt to help, put me in touch with another student who had also been very ill at university. I remember the awkwardness of our meeting, my attempts to radicalise her, to introduce her to the anger she must surely feel about her treatment and the society we were both a part of, and her bemusement. Her tale of her experience of psychosis and a diagnosis of schizophrenia and how life was hard but she was coping and hoping to finish her degree and move on. It made me uneasy. I had more or less given up on university, or the path people like me usually took in life, and did not like her acceptance of what was happening to her. It was only many years later, when I realised that being sectioned on a number of occasions had kept me alive too, that I began to understand her viewpoint.

Fast forward to my arrival in the Highlands, after a stint of setting up advocacy groups and working with Patients Councils in Lothian and elsewhere. I was still fascinated by Asylum magazine, excited by the Trieste model, scandalised by the idea of community treatment orders, convinced the voice of people with a mental illness was the purest, the most important. I was still sure that carers (in other words, my mum and dad – even in my early thirties!) had little right to speak about our treatment and that everything about the mental health system was about the uneven and abusive use of power in our treatment.

However, meeting people in different settings: the old asylum of Craig Dunain, (still occupied by many patients) church halls and drop-in centres in different villages across Highland, I found something very different to the debate of the cities. We were still angry about how people with a mental illness were treated but it seemed to be a more genuine anger somehow. You didn't need to have experienced a crash course in the theory of oppression; there was no requirement to be a committed socialist to want to have a voice. You didn't have to sneer at any community services set up by faith-based organisations. What people talked about was based on people's first hand experience. It seemed real, heartfelt, not something they had been taught to say or believe.

The very first thing we decided to talk about was what would happen to our old asylum now that it was being shut down. I already knew! Hospitals were, by definition, bad, and if sited in old Victorian buildings on the edge of town, even worse. The people who I was working with to create a new voice for our community told me something different. They said that that hospital had saved their lives; that many of the staff were almost friends. That they loved the woods and the views, the duck pond and the old graveyard. That it was often a place of peace and privacy and mutual support and that there was no way that they hated the idea of hospital and no way that they wanted to be treated in the centre of the town. We used their arguments with the health board and 'won' the point and my perspective changed.

It set me on a new path. The direction I had been taking, where my viewpoints were an article of faith from whoever was the latest guru in our movement, fell away, to be replaced by the need to gather the grass roots voice of our community, eventually to realise that contribution and change did not have to be a battle. That many of the workers we associated with shared our views and wanted us to succeed in our vision of a better world for us all.

Over the years, way up in the very north of the country, we wrote reports involving hundreds of people, worked with government, councils, health boards, the police; went into schools where we spoke with thousands of children, educated professionals, made films, appeared in the media, held art exhibitions and gave spoken word performances. Made, for a time, a huge difference in services, policy and the law. We attracted the attention of European partners and found ourselves in Romania and Catalunya, Portugal and Poland. We realised that partnership, kindness and dialogue and giving the benefit of the doubt was usually the best and most pleasant way of creating change.

I returned to the Central Belt of Scotland six years ago and, with my memoir published, discovered, very late, the debates, arguments and passion of mental health Twitter and the prominent national voices, of which I now seem to be a part. I became aware of an international movement that bewilders me in its bitterness. I now find myself confused by aspects of the movement I have spent much of my life with. Sometimes there is so much anger, such confrontation! It dismays me. I meet people who, desperate for their own vision, will do whatever they can to force their point forward. They don't care if they damage other people in the process. They don't give a jot for the evidence about what does and doesn't work. If, in their need to win, they send fellow people with mental illness back into despair that is just collateral damage. To think that many professionals are natural allies, or a manager has good motives, is laughable even to some of the more moderate members of the fashion for an organised voice we have nowadays. Managers are responsible for our deaths, psychiatrists know nothing of our worlds and have no possibility of empathy; are not worth speaking to unless they come prepared with apologies. It makes me terribly sad.

I remember with fondness those times in Highland when we could be in an operational meeting, planning services, and because we took the trouble to get to know each other, I knew that about eighty percent of the professionals present had also had mental health problems themselves. I remembered our own meetings in the north where support workers,

CPNs and, occasionally, psychiatrists joined in and shared their own experience of mental illness and were welcome.

Sometimes, I find my loyalty divided when I hear someone calmly and sensitively sharing the evidence of what leads to a reduction in restraint or seclusion and all I can hear is the blinkered response, "This is not good enough. It has to stop completely and immediately!" Sometimes, I despair a little when my fellow people with lived experience say, "I don't mind the effect of what I say. This is my passion, this is my right. As someone with lived experience, I have the right to speak as and how I want to. It is up to you to deal with how I come across!"

And sometimes, when I hear people saying, "Those managers, they earn a fortune, they don't know our world, they do not care at all." I know that many of those very managers start work at seven in the morning, finish after seven in the evening; work weekends, feel the same despair we do, take the same antidepressants we do; crave time with their children and their friends and partners in the same way that we do.

Then I wonder at my own path; the consequences of my voice and my fellow peers' voices over the years. Sometimes I crave the chance to sit down and talk, to share a meal, to go for a walk. Anything other than engage in the politics of division that I thought I had left behind thirty years ago, when I first went to the Highlands and found a different way of finding out and acting on our common collective voice.

September

2021—SEPTEMBER—WENDY—BOWLING AND THE FORTH AND CLYDE CANAL

Beside the canal there are so many bulrushes. I have very rarely seen bulrushes in much quantity. The air is still but there are no midges. Sometimes, as we walk along, little fish come to the surface, leaving round circles of ripples and the sudden slight swirl that attracts us to start with.

Wendy finds bushes full of sloe berries but doesn't know what they are. I think maybe I should come back to collect them to make sloe gin. She does know what the brambles are, of course, and pauses every so often to pick them and eat them. She is on a mission to stop me walking in front of her which to my shame I have to admit I do all the time.

An ideal day, the hint of rain, but only just. It doesn't fall. Cuddles and giggles in bed in the morning; later, me and Dash in the park where I read my book while sitting on a bench while Dash got confused by the fact that we weren't walking.

Walking along the Clyde among the trees in Bowling. Those two intertwined apple trees, one with red apples and one with green. I think they are crab apples but am told no, they are the eating type. The faint smell of woodsmoke from fires from the night before. The crows and seagulls on the mud of the beach. The waves from a tug that has passed on its way down the Clyde.

Encounters with dogs and their owners, the smell of Himalayan balsam which Wendy has grown to dislike. Remember that labrador that was so shy it couldn't wag its tail but clearly wanted to play with Dash? Or the spaniel that looked so mournful?

I can't remember a word of what we talked about that day, but there was indeed a lot of talking. You could call the words inconsequential but they are the opposite of that, they are the web that binds us together, the music of our walk by the water.

And that bowl of split pea soup when we finished! Dash tied to the table, yearning to play with all the other dogs, us sipping our soup, eating our toasties. Going home with a cheesecake in a tub to eat later with our coffee. I wish every day was like this!

2021—SEPTEMBER—MY JOURNAL

I met my dad again in my dreams, a different one this time. We were all in the Caribbean in bright sun, lots of blueness and sparkly water, lots of white buildings. I was closing down my dad's businesses but cannot really remember why. I remember my mum was very grumpy, especially with Dad.

I suppose that must mean something or other, he hasn't been back since then. Maybe we are finally leaving each other. It is strange, my memory is always of his face when it was very, very brown. Maybe in his seventies, certainly when he still seemed relatively healthy and spent so much of his time in the garden.

This September, the days are definitely much shorter, not a trace of daylight when I take Dash out in the evening. The toadstools are out, the geese are here, bobbing on the water, being noisy. The last few days were pretty grey and dull but there have been so many bright and sunny ones too. It's strange to think that a few years ago we were absolutely exhausted from all the weeks visiting Sandy in hospital and yet for the last three days we have spent so much time relaxing. I have got up late, we have been out walking, getting Wendy ready for her Kilt Walk, then back home, watching *Good Girls* on the telly before we both go to our separate beds to relax. That freedom, when free of the children, to lie in bed listening to the radio, sleeping, not even thinking of writing or reading, just doing nothing much. My work for September has died down hugely, no more long hours with the review or stuff like that.

I could be reading up on stuff, being more active, making sure I keep earning, but knowing I have some free days is such luxury and such a relief.

Just now I am upstairs while Wendy welcomes yet another new worker to work with her. Dash will be somewhere downstairs as he has gone off sleeping upstairs with me. That is a strange feeling. I still tread carefully when I get out of bed at night to go to the loo, trying to avoid stepping on him, only to remember he now sleeps downstairs. At the moment all the blinds are drawn, there is just the glow of the lamp, the sound of *Woman's Hour* and the rooks in the trees.

I had a strange few days recently, when I suddenly saw myself in a new light. I became acutely aware of, or believed I was acutely aware of the fact that most people despise me. I suppose I have said this before but it wanes and grows all the time. It was a horrible period that is still here to an extent. I saw myself as arrogant, confrontational, convinced of my own importance and ideas, this pompous, opinionated person, sure he is superior to everyone else. This was how I decided the people around me saw me. It makes me very unhappy and very confused when the moorings of how I see myself can shift around so spectacularly. I don't know many people well, really, and so don't quite know how it is that they actually see me. Wendy tells me that I am gentle and kind. I hope I am but really do not have a clue. I wonder whether this happens much to other people, a sudden loss of confidence in your identity?

I am not sure what is happening this month. We are just easing into autumn, the leaves are turning. I am having to start thinking of jumpers and coats again, of starting the mornings again in darkness.

I have had more commissions to do: writing workshops and articles. That feels good. I wish I could do more than that. I carry on going to

Jean's Bothy which is lovely. To feel relaxed there and in the company of people I trust is such a relief.

I have a few speeches to give but not much is happening at work, it seems to be happening with everyone else, but for me, I am not particularly busy and for some reason not particularly bothered that I am not busy. I seem to have stopped being consumed with the need to prove anything or do anything much. Ideally, I would just read books, go for walks and sleep.

I have no idea why this is how I am just now. I wish I could be collecting brambles and other berries, making jams and bottles of gin liquor. Maybe I will get some more energy in coming days.

It is a contrast to just a few years ago. Then, we were so fed up with eating quick meals out before going to visit Sandy in hospital but equally, when he got home and stopped treatment, determined to do things even if only so we could cheer Sandy up on our daily visits. I remember that promise we made, that those last few months would be as good as we could make them, not the terrible time that Sandy was so worried they would be. They were good; we had fun. A strange way of putting it, but we did.

2021—SEPTEMBER—ALAN—FATHERHOOD

I paused just now, slightly astonished as I found I was unsure what I would say about my dad in this chapter. With that astonishment, I realised much of my stories about my dad are not of Alan Morgan but my perspective of him from when I was a child; my perspectives of his fatherhood.

It made me think I would spend a short time in this small section talking about fatherhood. This also makes me pause! I am 58 and could not explain fatherhood to myself, let alone you.

Why do we not have those conversations as a routine? Why do we not talk about them at school? Why is there an absence such as this in our education? A gap before we become parents? We arrive, fresh-dreamed with scanty, optimistic ideas of what we will do for our children. For some of us, there is a promise not to give our children the childhood we had. I think both my dad and I had that in our minds.

I have just realised that in all the years I knew him, I never had a conversation with my dad about parenting. I had a lot of conversations blaming him for his parenting of me, which he put up with remarkably well, but not one where I asked for advice or just talked about being a parent and not one where he offered his advice or just talked about it.

I wonder what we would have learned if we had dared have that conversation? I think in his later years we might have given each other such a hug and said,

"We got it so wrong and we really did not mean to!"

I have been giving talks to a perinatal mental health network about my early fatherhood. I talk about the sheer terror I felt at becoming a dad. There was so much I did not know and so much I feared. When my wife became pregnant she felt incredibly sexy; I felt the opposite. Our baby was in there, how could we have sex?

I worried I would get it all wrong. I worried about everything. Yes, of course I was delighted, but so frightened. Could I do this? How would our life change? Would he really feel loved? Would my wife carry on loving me? Would we still do fun things?

The trivia of how to change a nappy, burp a child, calm it when it is crying through the night, coo love songs to it, carry on working. Find things for it to do. Not sit with my eyes drooping, early mornings when he is playing in the sitting room and I am meant to be entertaining him and have not a clue how to and have not a clue how to keep my red-rimmed eyes from shutting in those blessed moments of silence.

I told the nurses and health visitors I was teaching about that. I told them that when they see us dads with our awkward attempts at confidence and whatever it is, not to dismiss us. However much this parenting seems to be the province of our partners, I told them to recognise the exhaustion, the need we have to seem together and with it and how, for some of us, the opposite is the case; that far from looking after our new family, we are sinking deeper and deeper into something unmentionable.

At the same time as telling the midwives my story and how, a scant five months after my son was born, I was locked away in hospital on a section, I was also writing a short story: 'Failed fatherhood in approximately three and half thousand words.'

It is truly awful! But I thought it was good while I was tapping away at my laptop. It was influenced by some poems by Aoife Lyall, which truly moved me. In my few thousand words I talk about my trips to hospital, my son's numerous struggles with education, and life when he was a child and the finale, when he said he never wanted to see me again.

I would really love to sit down with my dad; not when his words were slow and he had to pause to consider them in his later years but when he was alert and yet prone to some self-reflection.

I would love to know what he felt when he was on constant standby to fly his jet fighters to intercept Russian bombers and I and my brother were at home being looked after by our mum. I would love to know how much he saw of us; if he changed our nappies or talked nonsense to us with a grin on his face. I would like to tell him that on the day my son was born I found it perfectly normal to spend the day at a conference I was running while my wife waited to go into labour after her waters broke. I would like to say,

"You know how I wanted to share the care of my son fifty-fifty with my wife? Both of us working part time? Really, I felt some relief when it became clear my wife didn't want to go back to work and loved my son so totally that the thought of me giving up any of my hours seemed silly. I just didn't know what to do. I didn't know how to charm or entertain him. I fell back into work with a sense of deliverance. Did you feel the same?"

I do wonder. I think that maybe a dad in the 60s would not have thought anything else, that it would have been extraordinary for him to share the childcare, but I wonder if he ever felt a regret that he didn't and so didn't develop the bonds that we did with our mother. Instead, he was the man we sometimes saw at breakfast, staring wide-eyed at him in his uniform while he ate his breakfast. Or he was the man who made us go for walks on the weekend, or later, the man who made us cry with his longwinded explanations of things we never understood or the man we muttered about when he ordered us to do things a certain way on the boat. Someone I started off in awe of, became afraid of, resented hugely and only much later, came to love.

I wonder what he felt about it? I know he had regrets. I have regrets too. I would love to have been able to tell my dad, "What idiots we were! You do realise, your regret at respecting my refusal to see you when I first tried to kill myself was misplaced? The damage was long done by then. It needed all those subsequent years of bitterness for me to see my own role in our mini tragedy."

I want to tell him, "I always regret that when my son said, 'Never speak to me again,' when he wrote that Post-it note saying, 'Fuck off,' when I wrote to him that I respected that and did not camp on the doorstep to our house, sure of his love, sure he would change his mind."

But of course, I was far too late by then too. I hope somewhere my dad can feel me saying sadly and maybe with the humour of admission, "I made just the same mistakes you did too and do you know why? I think I was too sure I was unloveable, unreachable. That I deserved every unshed tear that continues to scorch my memory. I think you were like that too, so much more vulnerable than I ever knew you were."

2021—SEPTEMBER—MENTAL HEALTH AND ME— LESSONS, SO LATE

Yesterday after school, while I was making tea, Wendy took wee Charlotte down into the forest walk where the bramble bushes are. Despite having an unopened jar of store-bought bramble jam, they both wanted to pick enough brambles to make their own jam.

Just as I was about to put the potatoes into the oven, the door opened and a wailing Charlotte tumbled in and rushed upstairs to the shower.

While she was picking the berries, she stood on a wasps nest and the furious insects poured out and flew up the inside of her trousers, stinging her. They stung her mum too, when she tried to rescue her. The shower was to get them off and out of her clothes.

They spent the evening taking antihistamines, with creams and cold packs pressed against their numerous stings.

This morning I came downstairs and put the coffee on and started making the children's lunch while Wendy clamped the downie over her head to get more sleep and Charlotte snuggled in, also grabbing the last remnants of the night.

While Wendy was drinking her coffee, I asked Charlotte what she wanted for breakfast but she only buried herself further under the downie. Wendy put her school clothes on the sofa bed and she curled even further under the downie and shouted from underneath that she wasn't going to school because of the wasps of last night.

After threats to phone her dad, threats to phone the school and say she was refusing to go to school, and a very teary Charlotte huddled in the sitting room, Wendy came to me in the kitchen and said she had changed her mind, that even Charlotte's brother, James, thought she should stay at home and what did I think?

For a brief moment, a flash of irritation crossed my mind, that flicker of, 'she shouldn't get away with it,' to be followed by the thought that it was horrible for her to be chased by the angry wasps and a relieved, "Yes, of course."

Her dad was kind when he heard of our drama about school but threatened to send homework through which made Charlotte smile. The headteacher had no problem with it either.

These events make me pause. I tend to cast back to my childhood for glimpses of what is right and wrong and know that as a child, the idea of my will overcoming an adult's would never ever have been an option. I reach for that knowledge and find it battles my own life now. I doubt I would ever have dared to challenge my parents or my teachers. I always felt their power was absolute. That memory hangs throughout my life now.

When the children are out of order, I tend to think they should not be allowed to get away with their behaviour, tend to think they should be sent to their room or punished, or at least say sorry.

Wendy has opened my eyes to the realisation that if they are out of order, outrageous even, that there is probably a good reason for it. She has shown me that gentleness, laughter, hugs and giggles may tease from them their worries, because there always are worries at these times, bursting to get out and find some little place of peace.

While Charlotte ate her Honey Loops in front of the telly next door, I emptied the dishwasher, tidied away the sofa bed and noticed my statement that I am meant to be signing and scanning and sending back to the police in the next couple of days.

I paused at that and remembered my shattered dreams from last night where I could not get comfortable and felt full of anxiety about how to live my life, approach my work, my family. It made me remember the last few weeks where I have had to fundamentally re-evaluate my character and how I think people see me; that shocked realisation that how I see myself may be totally flawed and the void in perception this is causing.

And with that, I remembered the discussion around suicide prevention. There is a book in my bookcase all about that and maybe one day I will read it, but just for the moment I think of Charlotte downstairs, probably drawing while vaguely watching *I Carly,* feeling safe and looked after.

I do not have the wit or the skill to know how to be an ideal parent and I have no idea what I would have needed in my growing up, or even if it would have made any difference in stopping my constant desire as an adult to cease to exist, but I am fairly sure that what I learnt as a child caused some of the insecurity that is such a part of my life.

For me, knowing the children feel safe enough at home to be rude and to swear and to challenge us; feel safe enough with their mum to cuddle up with her at night and talk about what has gone wrong at school. Happy enough and secure enough to make fun of me and, in the case of one, to give me great big 'I love you' hugs and, for the other to pretend to be mortally afraid that I will get too close to him while giggling all the time, paints a very different picture to the one I remember of my childhood spent mainly away from home, at school.

I am sure that love and kindness and warmth are far, far better than thinking I had to do everything adults ever told me to do; much better than worrying about that teacher whose idea of tenderness was anything but tender. Those crowded dormitories where it was better to keep private and silent, to hide emotion far, far away. Where it was important to seal the idea that you are loved, deep away from your consciousness, because what you are experiencing feels like anything but love.

It feels strange, now that I am approaching, or may already be in the middle of old age, that the ten-year-old twins are already more mature than I have ever been; that I could learn from Charlotte how to dare to give a cuddle back or from James how to risk rejection with some silly trivial action that I am too frightened to do just now.

To have found this family is wonderful. When there is no one in the house I still wander around it saying, "I want to die," but more and more I wish I were twenty, maybe thirty years younger, ready to find out just how wonderful life can be.

October

2021—OCTOBER—WENDY—THAT PAUSE IN A SMALL OASIS OF PLEASURE

Just as we were about to cross the road at the harbour in Eyemouth, I saw a quick swirl and the sleek black glistening back of a seal rising then disappearing in the water. It looked so powerful.

We paused, watched a fishing boat set off out from its moorings and then Wendy saw the swirl and gleam of the seal too and was delighted.

We ate in a pub: scampi for Wendy and fish and chips for me and, while we ate, talked to another family whose dog had fallen in love with Dash.

Leaving the pub, we saw more seals, closer than either of us have ever seen them before. We were both even more delighted.

From the end of the harbour we watched a collie dashing along the edge of the beach; racing the waves and always getting soaked at the end of its run. It looked so happy.

I am made for days like these!

Our Airbnb is wonderful; we had booked it to take the kids on holiday but found out that they were due at their dad's parents at the same time and instead of cancelling, decided on 'us' time for a couple of days.

It has been amazing. A drive through fog and rain, spray everywhere. Headlights, the constant sweep of the wipers, not totally sure where we were going.

Winding down a narrow lane in Reston, a sudden tight turn over a railway bridge and there was our cottage. It has a wonderful kitchen made of reclaimed wood, a woodburning stove we never lit, a sofa bed downstairs in front of the telly, all made up. Below that floor is a narrow room that leads to a conservatory which would be the ideal place to sit and write. Upstairs, in the eaves, is a double bedroom with windows looking out on one side to trees and a valley and the other side, up a hill to fields with sheep in. Next door to that, a clean, sparkling bathroom.

Arriving, I made a pot of coffee, after I had tidied away and took it, along with the croissants that had been left out for us, to Wendy, who was already curled up in the sofa bed, watching telly. For someone who uses words for a living, I can't describe properly how wonderful the next few hours were. Somehow, being officially on holiday seemed to release a switch in each of us. Snuggled up, lots of talking, even me talking! Bits of leg tangled in each other, elbows occasionally getting on hair. Dash curled up on the solitary chair at the other side of the room. The curtains drawn. A treasure land to remember the possibility of relaxation and warmth and company; a long drawn out sigh of, "This is just what we needed!"

An evening together; making dinner; vaguely watching telly. Time for us to do nothing but enjoy the company of each other. It feels like years since we have just luxuriated in each other's presence. Bound up in sleep and caresses and kisses. Silly stories; gulps of wine, crunchy hula hoops and freedom from all the pressures of the world.

Imagine if we could have this all the time. No pressure from work; all our stresses and worries swept away. Oh! It would be so wonderful.

I don't need reminded how lucky I am; these short moments are all I could ever need.

2021—OCTOBER—MY JOURNAL

I have come to write of October and cannot find my memory of it from the very beginning of the month. I think it involved rain and wind, dead leaves, more toadstools, lots of geese and the occasional bat and Wendy's daft but hopefully inspired idea to foster another labradoodle puppy.

On Saturday I came down south to see Mum for the week. After some frantic organising, we are all going to be here together: that is, Mum and her 'children', to finally scatter Dad's ashes.

My train journey was so long. I really did not want to read 'Restrictive practices in health care and disability settings' and I didn't want to read something enjoyable or to write. I didn't even really want to eat much of the lunch I made the day before. I closed my eyes a lot and felt glad that it was not terribly uncomfortable wearing a mask.

It has been good to see Mum; the weather is warm here but Mum says it is cold. There are flowers still out in her garden.

We went up to Firle the first day I was here. There was the strangest atmosphere; just a light wind, grey skies and in many places the haze and mist of drizzle. That silence and softness that nevertheless has sound, that closed-in-ness but at the same time breaks in the murk so we could look down on the Sussex villages and fields. There were paragliders drifting off the edge of the Downs, horses ambling very slowly, while their riders talked passionately to each other. There were dog walkers and families and us. I very much enjoyed it.

We are not having earnest conversations about Dad, which in a way is lucky as I do not have the confidence or skill to go there and keep having to stop myself from asking blunt questions, like:

"Are you lonely?"

"Do you miss him?"

I did ask if she thought he had had a good life and that pleased her because she genuinely thought he had had just the life he wanted, apart from the last few years of his illness.

I went to church for the first time since the funeral. I still feel very awkward and wrong going into churches but Mum wanted to go for the 'quiet time' and wanted my company and Arwen, the Reverend, had, some time ago, taken away some of my fear of churches and what I might do to them by my presence.

St Peter's is a very beautiful small church. I sat in the pew, itching my nose through my mask, trying to think about Dad; realising that my assumptions of our mutual failure with children is a bit off. I think if my illness is real, it colours my memory a little; makes it harder for me to see the brightness and lightness of childhood that was certainly there, despite some of the real darkness that existed. I wish I had a sort of ready-made video that could bring to life picnics or dog walks, or camping trips, or the memory of my parents singing as we drove places or that lovely cosy safe feeling when we slept in the back of the car on long night time journeys home from holidays.

My phone rang in the middle of 'quiet time'. It was on vibrate but still everyone heard it and that plunged me into all sorts of other thoughts; of my brother and of Jess and wondering if her operation had gone ok and of my sister and how on earth she will fit in everything when she gets here and how Keri is doing.

When I woke this morning, it was from the frantic memory of a dream of work gone wrong. I woke sweaty and anxious and exhausted and felt grateful to Kirsty for suggesting that I don't do any work for the review this week: to get a proper break even though I won't get paid. It is a good and sensible idea, despite the amount of reading I need to do to catch up on our program. I also woke determined to try to spend time away from alcohol. Initially I thought maybe I should stop drinking completely but being more realistic or maybe totally unrealistic, I think I might try later in the month to have weekdays drink free . I hope I manage it.

The day before, we were sitting in the kitchen, getting ready to go out when Mum said that this time two years ago she would have been sitting at the same table while Dad was dying in the hallway. We hastily went walking at Altringham Reservoir, which I have never been to before but one they both loved going round, and it was lovely. A bright blue sky, lots of birds, mainly gulls, and an hour or so's wander. Mum and I tease each other and laugh a lot nowadays, which I like. It somehow seems tender and somehow seems to stop the need for unnecessary confessions.

I do wonder how she will react to this book. Everyone knows it is being written and no one has objected, but I am sure that Mum would be terribly upset if I said terrible things about Dad and that Richard is already storing up worries; for someone whose job is about the harshest inner worlds anyone experiences, he is remarkably keen not to bring them into the open in the family which I think might be wise. I still don't think he could bring himself to do much more than skim read *START* despite it now being three years in print. When I am finished I will have to re-read these words to get perspective when I send what I will think is complete and precious, to them for comment.

We went out the next day, to walk to the wetlands along the beach and then across the new bridge at Tide Mills. Mum had been saying it was a beautiful day and that we must be out so I gobbled breakfast and we set off.

Just as we were saying what a wonderful walk we were having and how good the day was going to be, Mum stumbled when I had turned away to take a photo. She catapulted forward and dunted her head on the path. We sat together for a bit on the gravel and concrete and she gathered her thoughts and realised she was not hugely injured, but injured nonetheless.

Two ladies came up who were very kind to us, checking to see if Mum was ok, checking whether she was dizzy, pointing out errant drops of blood. They helped me get Mum on her feet and luckily I ignored her suggestion that I finish the walk alone while she made her own way home, and we went back. We knew her thumb was bleeding a lot but couldn't work out where the other blood on her hand was coming from, and we knew that her knees and elbow were bleeding because they hurt and had stuck her clothes to her. Occasionally I would dab at her eyebrows where the skin was also split, with blood running into her eyes.

By the time we got to the car, even Mum agreed that it was good to go home. Our initial idea was to go home, get her showered and settled down for the rest of the day. But when I realised how difficult she was finding it to get in the car, I suggested the doctors. Mum was saying, "I hope I don't become one of those old ladies who fall over all the time," while bits of her clothing were being spattered with red droplets.

In the house, I helped her take off her shoes and then her fleece and, once upstairs, her shirt. Once I saw her grossly swollen elbow, I told her that we were definitely going to take her for some help. Initially she said there was no problem but then she too saw it in the mirror and agreed.

We ended up at Lewes Urgent Treatment Centre. They were extremely nice to us. We got parked and seen very quickly and three hours later a bandaged Mum got back in the car and we went home.

Mum was determined to make light of her injuries and I was determined to make sure Richard and Juliet knew that Mum really was quite damaged when they arrived.

The days since have been lovely; only two of them but it has been gentle and pleasant. Jess has had her op and is bound in a sling and doing ok. Juliet arrived with a cut nose and a black eye because when she was in Somerset, Frodo the dog found a huge vase which he managed to put his head in and get stuck in. In his panic at being trapped, he smashed the jar, leaving himself with a collar of jagged glass, and in their efforts to free him and end his panic, Juliet got headbutted by his glass collar, hence the injuries. It all seems a bit dramatic just now!

I do not know how to describe these days; lots of reminiscing and laughter, lots of, do you remember? And did this happen? And who was this? And what photo is this of? Lots of gentleness.

Richard has been very funny and very generous. Making us a huge paella, doing his deadpan unemotional thing which both is and isn't put on. I am so glad to have been in his company. He makes me realise how much I love him, wish that I could speak with him in the way he probably would like me to, rather than in the ways I don't dare to and know he would hate. I have spent more time with Jess than ever before which has been brilliant; just learning bits of her life, about her partner, the job she will have in the Caribbean when her arm is ok, in about three months time. She is a tender girl and quite astonishingly beautiful and what is lovely, is to see how much she loves her dad. And Juliet is as ever, the lovely Juliet.

After a mammoth search for a container for Dad's ashes we realised what it was already in was just fine.

The night before, I put it on the table in my room, wrapped in its RORC flag, with pictures behind it of sailing boats and fighter jets. There really should have been family pictures but this seemed apt too. I held Juliet for long moments while she cried and then left her to light a candle and sit with Dad while I went downstairs for whisky.

Today was the day we took Dad to sea...

We arrived early, to the sound of a freighter being filled with scrap iron. I had Dad's ashes in their box, wrapped in the flag, alongside Richard's bottle of Laphroaig. Jess couldn't decide whether to come with us in case the ride was bumpy and messed up her shoulder again but Paul the boatman said the sea should be very smooth.

I remember Mum getting into the boat with some difficulty and how it was kept on a sort of floating dock.

Juliet and I were up near the bows while Mum, Jess and Richard were in the stern. The sea did its usual silver glittering thing and was very still, if sea can ever be still. I had chosen the Jupiter sections from Holst's *The Planets* as a choice of music to listen to on our way because I remembered sometimes Dad played it very loud on Christmas Day. Paul connected it to his sound system, it was loud and a bit thrilling.

Once we were past the kittiwakes and the confines of the harbour, we zoomed along, close to Seaford beach. To be at sea again after all these years was wonderful, to see Seaford and the Seven Sisters from this perspective, brilliant.

We cut the engine off of Splash point and drifted on the waves. Juliet and Mum read from a reading, Juliet lit frankincense in a bowl and a haze of fragrant smoke wafted over the water. I unwrapped Dad's ashes and began to pour them into the sea; finally having to take the packet out of the bag to finish the job and, somewhat to my satisfaction, getting a slight dusting of Dad on my hands. Juliet threw flowers from the garden into the sea. Mum wished Dad a good journey among the oceans he loved. Richard poured us each a tiny measure of whisky and then a measure for Dad that he poured into the sea. We had some quiet time.

Mum couldn't finish her whisky so Richard gave Dad the rest of her measure too.

I think we all felt a little hint of tears at this time. We were gladdened when a sailing boat passed close by us, almost symbolic in its arrival.

Then, not much more than an hour later, we were ashore and went to the pub that Dad often used to take us to: The Ox near Alfriston where we drank one of the beers Dad always liked to have.

Both Mum and I tried to pay for the lunch but Richard insisted that he paid. He is so continually generous to people. It is good to see.

We played Scrabble in the evening. I had said I wouldn't play as I don't like such things but in the end Jess made me help her as she said she needed a reasonable adjustment for her dyslexia. It was an evening full of laughter and that was how it should be.

It was so good to do as Dad wished and lay his ashes in the sea. I don't know if it has given a sense of completion but it was a good thing to do and a healing thing to do. I had been wondering if it would mean that I would no longer meet Dad in my dreams but last night he was there. He was in one of his outrageous moods and said that he had got two tests for Covid and that he now had had Covid twice over and that he had no intention of stopping working or isolating. I can almost imagine that side of him too. It is good to remember that as well.

Now I am home again, busy with work.

I got a lovely letter from Mum. She said in it how desperately she misses Dad. The sparse small words were so powerful because she does not usually say such things. They made my eyes prickle and reminded me of all those years they lived together, all that they went through and now she is alone and that makes me very sad.

2019—OCTOBER—ALAN—WHEN THE FABRIC TEARS

It might seem silly but I have often wanted to write a book or see a film where a family does things: nice things, boring things, little adventures and romances and disputes. A nice amble of a film where you are feeling warm and slightly pleased that you are watching it and then the family gets in the car, maybe to visit an aunt or their parents and, as they are driving along another car pulls out into their path and they are pushed into the other side of the road into the route of an incoming car and everything explodes. There is screaming and blood and noise and rubbish everywhere and suddenly that is it; that is the end of the film or the book because all the main characters are dead and or soon to die.

I would like that because it is so like life. Life's adventures and tragedies are so random; some things are expected but others just happen and that is that. The end. No moral, no tying up of loose ends, just the sudden jerk into something different, something completely different. Something final.

What were the months after Sandy died like? Wendy was getting back into the world again, more and more into the world.

We were planning holidays, or at least Wendy was, and doing much more visiting. Seeing Peter and Sharon's family, Sharon's sister's family, Juliet and David in their new house, all these things. There were also tiny things; we had taken two tubs of salt from Sandy's house which seemed a pity to throw away. I was watching them slowly empty, wondering how I would feel when I threw the last empty one away.

The children were flourishing, doing well at school, having sleepovers and play dates, going swimming, to football and the Brownies. James seemed to be especially happy but Charlotte was also getting there now she had a packed lunch, so that she could spend her lunch break with her best friends. She had less meltdowns, had fewer moments crying with her mama about her papa. Was writing amazing poetry, doing her crafts, getting, like James, obsessed with Pokemon and into Minecraft and Fortnite…

We had decided that I would visit my mum and dad every three months or so and that when I visited, then Mum could go to visit Richard or Juliet or do something for herself while I stayed with Dad.

I had been down already so that Mum could see Juliet, I think in her new house. I remember they did lots together: spent a day at Portavadie Marina, getting spoilt, wandering around Argyll, having fun.

And then, when was it? Late August/early September? I went down again so that Mum could go to see Richard's family.

I had a wonderful time with Dad. Mum had a wonderful time with them. Wendy came down a bit later and I so love how Wendy really liked Dad, just saw him as someone very special, and I was delighted that Dad really liked Wendy, joked with her, told her stories.

Those weeks were great. Richard and his family visited Mum and Dad after their amazing holiday in Canada. Mum and Dad's great friends, the Geoghegans, also came to visit them in September.

Juliet and all the children went down and had a great time. I was so pleased to hear, how, when Keri came in, she naturally just snuggled up between her grandad and grandma on the couch, was able to manage the conversation and keep it fun despite her grandad's lapses in ability to speak and organise his thoughts as he would like; was fine about some of his difficult moments. It sounded like a wonderful loving time for all of them.

October came and we were all needing a break, and we were going to get it because Wendy had decided long ago, before even her dad died, that this year we would have a special holiday to brighten up the last year, which had been so hard.

The children needed a break from school and us two from work. Everyone was very excited to be going to a village outside Disneyland and I was especially pleased that we would be going to other places as well as Disney during the week.

That holiday was lovely. I can see so well how much a difference it can be to get away to see the world with new eyes and encounter it with different feelings.

11 OCTOBER 2019—DEATH IN DISNEYLAND

I had a great time in France in our wee Airbnb with its grapevines, the boulangerie where every day, I bought baguettes and croissants and pain au chocolat. I loved the shop across the road with its piles of fruit, its tins and crisps, a multitude of different rums and wines. It was French. France! Exciting!

That first day when we woke up to the light after the late night arrival, I braved the rain and my lack of knowledge to walk into where I sort of thought the town centre might be! All those murals on the buildings, the Arabic shop owner who was so nice to me every day I went there. The fact that the shop was a gathering place; every evening there would be young men, mainly Arabian men, drinking coffee or beer and talking in the shop entrance and each time he was so kind to me, tried to say a few things in English, wished us well, helped tell us where to get the bus to Disneyland.

It would have been a good holiday, it still was a good holiday. First of all, a day of doing almost nothing because it was raining. All of us on the internet or reading, eating, drinking; me getting in the supplies of food, getting in the wine and whisky.

We went to Meaux the next day, anxious about how to get the bus, wondering which direction to travel in. Worried about where to get off and then wandering the streets, the very posh, rain-slicked streets, where we spent an inordinate time in Pokemon shops. Then the sandwich shop where I felt just like Dad must have felt when I saw him speaking in France when I was a child. There I was, busy trying to order our food in French, as the lady had no English and she burst out laughing, said she had no idea what I was trying to say and that I might as well have been speaking Martian! We all giggled a lot at that and then spent ages in the gardens by the cathedral, eating our lunch. There, the children tried to train the goldfish in the pool by the fountain which came out of a fern and moss-covered boulder. They decided that if they made the right gestures the fish would go where they wanted them to go!

The next day we were in Disney Studios.

We had an amazing time. We are a very cautious family so multiple rides on the whirling cars, the magic carpets, the slinky dog, were the main attraction for the children. But the very best was Ratatouille – breathtaking. We saved money by taking in our lunch and all the time the rain kept off, unlike the day before when we had got soaked to the skin on the way home.

The next day it was Disneyland again. James was terrified of Snow White on his very first ride. He clung tight to his mum, tried to have his hands over both his ears and eyes. Charlotte quite liked it, while James was dismayed by what he had seen; cuddled into his mum; scowled for the next hour or so, refused to go any rides until we went on the 'It's a

Small World' ride and were given a huge boat made for wheelchairs to ourselves and he was able to enjoy lounging around on it.

By the afternoon we were tired but had found a seat to sit and drink some water, next to a pirate ship and the Swiss Family Robinson tree house. We were very, very content, watching the people go by, sitting in the sun, contemplating fish and chips later, which, the last time we had them, the children insisted were chicken and chips.

Then my phone rang.

At first I thought it was one of those annoying sales calls until I noticed it was my mum's number.

I answered. Mum said Dad had collapsed and that he was being resuscitated but that it didn't look good and that she would call me when she had news.

I was brief, replying to her, assuming she had other people to call, wouldn't want lots of questions, would be busy with the hospital staff. Later, I found out that when she called, she was sitting in the kitchen while, in the hallway, the emergency services were busy trying to resuscitate Dad, who had had a heart attack in the downstairs toilet. I imagine she would have so much loved some comforting words as the paramedics rushed around, would have wanted a virtual hug in the knowledge she had, that Dad was probably already dead.

She told me later they were very respectful and did all they could for Dad and her, and that even though within a short time they knew he was dead, they still stayed another three hours until they were sure Mum was ok, tidied him up, did what they could. Left her to sit with him, to say goodbye to him and most importantly, told her that he probably didn't feel a thing or even know what was happening.

After that it was all a bit weird. At the time, I still didn't know Dad had actually died. Wendy tried so hard to comfort me, was so sure I would be in a mess but I wasn't. I wasn't thinking at all. Mainly I was thinking about whether I should go straight to England and leave Wendy to make her own way home with the twins. Thinking about how she would do so and how I would buy a ticket and what we would do about the car that needed picked up from the airport parking in Glasgow if I went to England instead.

We were organising, wondering whether I should go to the airport on the next train, wondering what to do. Wondering if Dad would recover, if my hesitation might mean that I would not see him for what might be the last few days of his life.

Charlotte gave me a huge, teary hug, Wendy gave me a huge hug too and James hung around the edge of us three, looking lost because he wanted to give me a hug too but has spent the last year saying he hates hugs from me.

He did say later on, privately to Wendy, that he would try to be nicer to me for the rest of the holidays.

We decided to carry on, by far the best decision. I texted Richard and Juliet and then Mum and we went to the play park where Wendy and I sat side by side against the walls and I don't know what we talked about. I think we talked about how, if he died this time, it would probably be far better than him having to face the relentless sapping of him that his Parkinson's was doing. That it might, in some ways, be a blessing.

The children dashed around, all excited for an hour, clambering up things, hiding from each other, chasing each other, inventing games. Then off to the tree house, then the suspension bridge and then finally off to Frontierland where, leaning against the fence for the paddle steamer, I got a text from Juliet where it was obvious that she didn't know that I didn't yet know Dad was already dead.

She said at least it was quick and painless. And then worried when I replied to say did that mean Dad had died?

I felt nothing, just felt a bit bewildered; knew that I didn't want to go to the fireworks later; found it funny when James said, "Why is Graham sad? Why does he need to go back to the house?"

When Wendy said I would be leaving them to see the fireworks alone, she had to say, "James, Graham's daddy has just died! Wouldn't you be sad if your daddy died?"

You could see confusion in his face because daddies don't die and then a dawning inkling in his eyes, some tears there at the enormity and sadness of it all. Tears that I didn't have.

My main preoccupation on the way home was to text Wendy times and bus stops for when she came home with the children in the dark.

At Montry, I went into the shop and bought one of the many bottles of rum. I think it was from Île de Réunion. (It was lovely, anyway. I never knew white rum could be so delicious.) I bought some crisps and nuts for when the children came home.

I wanted to tell the shopkeeper that my dad had died an hour or so ago, just as the next day, when they asked me how I was in the boulangerie, I wanted to tell them and when our landlords asked us how our holiday had been, I wanted to tell them, but for some reason we never did.

We never said our holiday was fractured. Instead, we just said we were having a great time, thanked everyone for being so nice to us.

Wendy came home earlier than we thought, with tales of hot dogs costing eight euros, of the fireworks. The children had been convinced she wouldn't find the way back. They tried to guide her in the right direction and on to the right bus and look after her. But she managed absolutely fine. I think it sometimes suits us to say we need to look after her, despite all evidence to the contrary and the glaring fact that she spends a large proportion of her life looking after us.

We stayed up late, all of us.

We munched on crisps, nuts and chocolate. I drank rum, the children went on the internet. We snuggled up and then I slept, not very well but not very badly.

I had drunk enough that I snored a lot, forcing Wendy to see if the children's bed was a better bet. It wasn't. There was no room for her. But somehow the noise I was making subsided when she got back and she was able to sleep too.

It was strange the next day, still on holiday but with a dead dad. We went back to Meaux. The children grumbled at all the walking but nattered to each other non-stop on the bus.

Once we were there we set off to find a café for lunch. The restaurants we encountered were all far too expensive for us to have a meal in. We walked through markets on bridges and on streets and under a huge shed. We looked at the cheeses, the clothes, the vegetables and ended up getting food from a boulangerie, eating at the tables of a locked up café.

Wendy kept on giving me hugs, asking me how I was and I kept on saying fine, but slightly dazed and slightly tired. I was very glad when Wendy said how hard it was when you wanted to give someone you love, comfort and at the same time know you can't really, that it won't change what has happened.

It reminded me of how incompetent I had sometimes felt when helping her with her dad.

The night before, Wendy had bought me train tickets to get to Mum's from Glasgow. We were relieved to know that Richard had gone down to her straight from work.

Somehow we were making silly mistakes. The tickets never came through, so she must have put down the wrong email address. Lots of silly mistakes for a number of days.

We worked out how to get to Crécy-la-Chapelle the next day. Me being anxious on the bus about where it would stop and keen to get back early to make our way to the airport.

Crécy really was the perfect place to go: a bright blue, hot, hot sky. Lots of canals with riverweed, flowers, people having meals at tables in narrow streets, people sketching, open air libraries, lots of dogs to pet. It took our mind off everything. It was now only every ten minutes that I was saying to myself, "My dad's dead." Feeling slightly astonished but mainly wondering what I was feeling or whether I was feeling.

And only every ten minutes that I didn't catch myself thinking about things we were doing he would have liked to have heard about and realising I would never be able to tell him about them.

Charlotte had been complaining of a spiky thing in her shoe and Wendy had been feeling her shoe, her socks, banging it upside down, time after time. Finally, I had a look and found a huge nail stuck to the undersole and felt delighted at the praise I was given. Charlotte was delighted too. Said, "See, I told you it was spiky."

Wendy was suitably apologetic, confessed that she was a terrible mummy.

Then we were back in Montry, picking up our bags; me happy that we had got the earlier bus to get to the train station and then the airport.

And then we were home, the children were at their dad's. I was eating pizza from the Co-op and we were contemplating the fact that the holiday Wendy had promised herself and the family as respite for her dad's death, eight months before, turned out to be the one when my own dad died.

She was right, though. I didn't know what it would be like. Sandy's death was sad and traumatic but my own dad's…? I don't understand what has happened. I don't know if I have any regrets for things unsaid, uncompleted. I don't know if I am sad. I don't know whether I am guilty that I am glad he will not suffer anymore. I don't know if I am relieved that Mum will not have that huge burden she had of looking after him anymore, or frightened for her future. The silent nights in a big house, all alone.

I don't know anything. I have had no revelation, no epiphany. There have been no cathartic words or the release of weeping. I still sleep better than I have for some months, but that is it, isn't it? I really, really do not believe Dad is dead.

It is like I am away at school and won't be seeing him for a time, or he just won't answer the phone on the Sunday phone call, not that he is dead. Not that I will never speak to him again, never hug him, never put the sun umbrella up for him in the morning and take it down in the evening. A whole litany of nevers.

*

This mourning or whatever it is that I am doing is so different to what I thought it would be. I am not in the slightest upset, not in the slightest. I regret that I will not be able to speak to my dad again, that he won't be sitting in the garden, reading, or asking me to open a bottle of wine at dinner or telling Wendy another of his stories, but really, I do not cry, I do not mourn.

But it does feel so physical, all of this. Just as though I have been in a huge fight or battle, as though I have walked a hundred miles and then been caught in a street riot. But only at times. Sometimes my throat is closed with anxiety, sometimes my stomach is hollow, like I might be sick, but so often I want to just sleep and stare, and not have to do anything with anyone.

The funeral went perfectly. First the crematorium and then the memorial service at St Peter's, the church my parents go to. We had done all the organising, sorted who would get the hall ready, how we would get to the crematorium, all that. And then there we were. I took Mum, Wendy, Keri and Finn in the car and I don't remember much of the drive, except that in the back they were all talking away.

There was no parking at the crematorium but luckily we managed to find somewhere on the street. I got a call, all panicky, from Juliet, thinking she had driven to the wrong crematorium, which she hadn't.

And then we were making our way to the family chapel, having to skirt the crowd of people who had been in just before us, lots of people with lots of flags and uniforms.

We did not quite know what to do but found Arwen who showed Mum and I the inside of the chapel and asked if we wanted to follow the coffin in or wait inside. Mum wanted to wait inside, so after Juliet and some of the girls had been to the toilet that is what we did.

I liked the coffin, when the funeral people took it in. All dark, with Dad's Royal Ocean Racing Club flag draped over it and that huge lovely spray of flowers.

And then it was singing which I didn't do, and which Richard did, slightly to my surprise. It was hymns and prayers. Fin read 'To the Lighthouse' by Virginia Woolf and Richard came up to speak. He could hardly speak, kept on having to dab tissues at his eyes. He was funny and loving and sad and terribly, terribly moving.

When his voice broke when he said he hoped that Dad knew he loved him, I could hear people behind me crying.

And then Juliet and David, Ella, Aran and Fin sang the Celtic Grace, gathered around the coffin, slightly halting at first. In the silence that followed, Juliet rested her head on Dad's coffin, making it bang loudly.

Holy water was sprinkled, blessings made and the curtain drawn around Dad.

When we were leaving, Mum stopped in front of the curtain and leant into me and said, "He really has gone now, hasn't he?" Gave a sob and said, "Goodbye, my love."

And at that I felt the first touch of a tear in my eyes. We had a hug and we walked out, off to the cars and home.

In the front of the car, we said nothing much, in fact Mum nearly fell asleep. She was so still and silent I reached out while driving to check she was ok. In the back, everyone was subdued and ended up talking about expressing emotion, talking about masculinity and how it is not always a sign of toxicity when men don't automatically cry when sad things happen.

At home, Richard was ever so organised, taking the young people to the chapel where Jackie (a friend of Mum and Dad's) had the food, along with the collage of photos of Dad.

Richard and the others came back just as the soup we were heating up was ready and Juliet and her crowd, just after.

We ate, I wandered around, impatient for us to start, and then we were walking down the road to the church: me, Mum, Wendy, Keri and Finn, with the others following further back.

Just as we reached the church, we found the Geoghegans and the Davidsons. Hugs and introductions and conversation until me and Mum moved away to the church.

Mum chose to sit by the wall in the front pew beside some flowers. Everything looked lovely; so many people, so many flowers and Arwen and two other ministery-type people. They walked down, following a cross, bowed in different directions, signed the cross over their chests; seemed more like Catholics than C of E people.

I was preoccupied, wondering if I would cry when I did my eulogy and knowing I wouldn't and worried about the devil stuff. Worried that by being there I was bringing evil into a holy place, worried that the congregation would fall into misery, the church burn down. I found it hard to believe that goodness could overcome my evil as Arwen had said happens, found it hard to believe that she could be right that I wasn't evil.

I didn't sing, stared at the floor. I didn't want to ruin something beautiful by trying to join in. As Arwen did her stuff, I seemed to be in a battle, trying to shrink my evil; sort of trying to explode so that the evil went and goodness overcame the darkness of me. It felt that if I contracted who I was as much as possible, it would reach a point at which the evil could no longer shrink and that then my evil would vanish and my new essence expand and somehow goodness would overtake everything.

I thought if that happened, I might have a heart attack too and worried

212

about the effect on the people around me. Wondered if that would be a sign of evil too.

And then I did my speaking and it went well and the church didn't fall down and I didn't feel anything. It was like any performance that I have done when telling sad and personal stories.

Peter read out 'Crossing the Bar' wonderfully. He has the most incredible voice but at the end that voice broke and he looked unsteady as though not sure he could walk back to his place in the congregation.

Juliet's eulogy was emotional and amazing. Wendy said the time she started crying again was when Juliet was talking about how safe she had felt when she had had her dad's big strong hand holding hers when she was a child.

The chapel for the after service was packed with people and looked beautiful, the 'children' all already there to hand out coffee and tea and wine. We four had been greeting people at the church entrance, but I can't remember much of what people said except that lots of them said my eulogy was lovely and could they hire me to give speeches?

And the chapel? Well, we talked, Peter sympathised at my hatred of small talk, I ate sandwiches and did manage to talk to various people. Keri came by with a big glass of wine and finally it was time to go home, carrying the leftovers, with two church people taking over the tidying for us.

I was tired, but we talked through the evening. Richard made a huge and lovely paella on his special portable paella pan and burner.

I think I tried to be funny a bit of the time. I think I was yearning for when we could go to bed without comment.

BLUE SKY MOURNING

I sat on my bed, my laptop on, the morning stretching ahead. Free time, a good sleep and I couldn't. I just couldn't.

I don't know why but it seemed better to stare into space, to fall into a dwam than to seize the chance to write. I do not think about my dad much now, it is not the ever-present reminder that it was for the first week. But it is strange. All of this is strange.

When my mum called me down to help her put the gathered fallen leaves into the bin, I felt a slight sense of relief and a touch of guilt that she has carried on, just doing it all, just doing it all.

Today is the first day in ages that has been bright and sunny. A wonderful change, so much better than the dreich rain of last week where the greyness and that hanging dampness have done nothing to improve our mood. But today? Well, today is a good one.

We decided to go to one of the pubs that Mum and Dad used to go to, away off at Firle – The Ram. A sprawling place with lit fires and low roofs. And there, in between eating our fish platter together, we talked about how we felt. It is a relief in a way that we both have similar feelings. Mum says she just feels different, as though something has happened but she doesn't know what. As if she is on the edge of things, as if the world is a bit further away. She doesn't so much feel as feel numb, she doesn't feel but her stomach feels the way it used to do before an exam. And I feel much the same, as though there is a heap of nothingness in my soul, as though I will wake up at some point and understand but maybe I won't.

Her friends tell her this is normal, tell her that it will change, that at some point it will all become real and she will feel the full impact. I hope I don't. I don't particularly want that.

But she also said that there is a sense of relief. Dad had been so dependent on her and had never wanted to go out anymore. For the last two years she has left him alone only for the shortest of possible times, always rushing back, not because he asked it of her, but because she worried about him. Despite their love she had become trapped and exhausted.

She said that now she might be able to stay behind and chat after the Samaritans finishes, that she could go to friends, out for a meal, off to the cinema, or just get fed up with her own company, pack her bags and come to visit us, her children, and we both agreed that we had mixed feelings, that maybe this death was a blessing. That it brought to an end what was beginning to be a very difficult life.

I liked that pub, our smoked salmon, our mackerel paté, the waitresses who seemed so friendly, the fire.

We carried on afterwards to the top of the South Downs, to Firle Beacon.

On a day like this they are beautiful. So green and smooth, the soft hollows and curves, the green, green grass and the dark shadows from the occasional cloud. The far off sea, shining bright silver with the dazzling sunshine. The dark shape of a ship leaving Newhaven. The bumble of light aircraft droning above us. Everything so still. The smoke far below, rising in a straight blue grey line from the occasional bonfire. The whistles of a man for his dog, the bleat of a sheep, the squawk of the crows.

It was lovely, and as we walked, we remembered times that I had walked with Mum from home to here in times past, when Dad could still drive out to meet us and take us home. I remember those times but they have become a bit too distant. I could not retrace our route from memory, I would need prompting. I cannot remember the conversations but I know that every time I went walking with Mum, Dad would have been part of what we talked about as we walked along the edges of the fields and up the gentle hills.

Mum mentioned the time, when Dad could still walk properly, when they went for a long walk up here. When they got back to the car, to go home, Dad patted his pockets and couldn't find the car keys. He decided that they must have fallen out of his pocket when he went for a wee behind a bush, some considerable distance away. Off they went to look for them, searched all around the bush, couldn't find them so they decided to walk home and, just as they were nearing home, Dad took off his jacket because he was hot and realised the light jacket he wore underneath had pockets too, in which rested the car keys! So, round they turned again, back to the car to take it home. Not much of a story but the sort of story that families remember. A "Do you remember that time when...?"

And now that is all we do have – memories of Dad. A strange feeling that I think I will take ages to get used to.

Work have been fantastic with compassionate leave. They were so strict about me not working at all while I was off, which feels very good.

2021—OCTOBER—MENTAL HEALTH AND ME— TRYING NOT TO LIVE—WHISKY AND ME

In *START* I mentioned alcohol and I think I had better mention it again. I do not understand my relationship with alcohol or that of some members of my family who also struggle with alcohol or drugs. When I say I do not understand; I really do not understand.

When Sandy died, he asked Peter to give me £1000 from his estate to spend on whisky, in recognition of some of the help I had given and of the fact that I do love a malt whisky.

I didn't buy much malt whisky with it but it did fund the considerable amount of alcohol I drink every day. My dad drank a lot, even up to not long before his death, despite reacting badly to it in the latter months.

Sandy almost never drank because his dad had drunk too much and not been kind with his alcohol and Wendy almost never drinks. I think because she just hates getting drunk and sees no point in it, maybe the fact that her gran died of cirrhosis played a part too. We both have friends whose relationship with alcohol especially, but sometimes with drugs, has taken them to the verge of death and has definitely caused the shattering of their relationships and lives and which we know will inevitably lead to their death and the tragedy that will cause to their families.

If I didn't drink so much I think I would despise our culture which seems unable to function without a drink, but then in the next sentence I think how funny Wendy, Sharon and Clare are after a drink, how much an evening seems to shine.

In contrast, I just fall asleep and become even quieter than usual. Since Sandy's death, three years ago, I have drunk about two litres of whisky a week, with some small exceptions. I don't even count the beer or wine that goes with it. My CPN is also an addictions CPN but we don't really talk much about my alcohol. I never tell her how much I drink and I only pay lip service to our joint plans for smaller measures and larger mixers and days off and later starts and earlier finishes.

If I know I cannot drink in an evening, for instance, if I am giving the family a lift, it is no problem, though I will look forward to a drink when we get home. I don't have any cravings and I don't feel bad when I don't drink but still I wish to drink.

The more I think about it, the more bizarre it seems. If this carries on I will die far too early for Wendy's family. It costs a fortune and gives me very, very little pleasure but it does dull my reality.

Sometimes over the last few years I have had alcohol-free months in response to Wendy's encouragement and when I do that I feel wonderful. I sleep better, have no fear that I may be over the limit if I drive early in the morning. I speak more and feel brighter but nowadays, the thought of a month without a drink, sends shivers into my thoughts.

I know drink is bad for your sleep but often it seems that with a drink I can actually sleep better and often it seems with a drink I can relax and I can stop thinking and I can put thoughts I do not want behind me. It feels like a cloak in which I can escape from my worst thoughts. To know I can fall into sleep within seconds of turning out the light; fall into sleep even though I keep the radio on and not have that agonised tossing and turning and worrying about almost everything. It is such bliss.

To find myself slow and soft in the evening seems to mean that I am not in any sort of 'doing' mode. I am not working or performing or trying to do anything. I am off duty from being me. I am free of the effort to meet any expectations. Having that marker that allows me to switch off is also bliss.

What is not bliss is that Wendy has grown to hate the smell of whisky on my breath, prefers not to have a kiss later in the evening. What is not bliss is that although switching off is indeed bliss, it is what it is: switching off, not being there for those I love. Not doing much more than watching the telly or posting on Facebook or Instagram. Not going for a walk or writing or making something. Not getting into a vibrant conversation, not staying up late, instead, waiting for that moment when I can go to bed without too much comment so that I can just sleep.

Sleep is such a haven for me. I hope that when I die that is what it will be like. To dive into nothingness feels like such privilege. My nights are my joy nowadays. I am either blissfully, delightedly absent or I am having dreams and they are often wonderful. In my dreams I meet my family: Wendy, my dad, the children, sometimes my son and it is more vivid and more real and always interestingly bizarre, and usually something I wake from in a good mood. Occasionally I descend into somewhere terrible but only rarely.

But I have early nights, Wendy has later nights. I have the radio on to tear away my thoughts, I snore so loudly no one can be near me. I have grown fat on alcohol. I sometimes stink of alcohol. We no longer lie side by side for hour after hour, talking and giggling. We no longer wake in the dark and turn to each other for a cuddle.

At work we are just about to start a series of interviews with people who have a dual diagnosis of substance abuse issues and mental illness. I am tempted to interview myself and some of the people in my life who are dear to me. I am tempted to say, just let me write this report, I know it inside out. But I don't.

I am nowhere near recovery. I have no desire to stop drinking and I cannot see any route out of it. Those brief moments where I have been treated for my drinking; those people seemed so judgemental and clinical, did nothing to help me want to make any sort of change in my life. I have always felt humiliated at those times and at the crude techniques they chose to try to get me to adopt.

In many ways I see my drinking as self harm, even as a slow suicide or even a type of living death in the absence I create of myself. When I wander the house saying, "I want to die," or find myself repeating it over and over again when walking Dash the dog or while driving the car, I can see alcohol as that answer.

And yet, despite this constant self destructiveness, my life is wonderful. I may be convinced I should be dead but when I walk downstairs and Charlotte surfaces from bed to give me a sleepy smile, or Wendy walks into the room in her dressing gown, ready for a hug and a kiss, or James says, "Woof woof" from his room or Dash stands on his hind legs to greet me, I know without doubt how lucky I am and how wonderful my life has become.

Whilst I want to die, I also want to live long enough to see the wee ones have their own children; to maybe hear from my son one day and to really learn how to love life in the way I glimpse every day and yet hide from every night when I hear the ragged break of the seal on the cap of the whisky bottle.

November

That word. It is soft, wispy. I can still imagine a wish being the fluff of dandelion blossom, drifting in the wind on the slightest of summer's breezes, bringing smiles and laughter and close-hipped cuddles.

I can also, now that the years have passed by me so many times, hear it as the delicate fall of leaves in the autumn when I take the dog out for his nighttime wee. That slight clatter in the forest as the rooks shift in their nests, the bats jink and flitter, somewhere the owls screech and elsewhere the foxes slink through the gardens.

I have no hesitation in saying what my wishes are but I have to qualify; to explain somehow and maybe, in the explaining, I will learn something for myself.

I am just back from walking Dash. As usual, we were at Ardmore. The day today was grey and windy and rainy. In the night the wind did that roaring sound in the gaps in the windows and Dash, for some reason, prowled through the house barking in the early hours until I got dressed and took him outside. But today I pulled down the hood from my waterproofs and let the wind and the rain onto my face and into my hair. My clothes rattled and the raindrops pattered. At the point, the cormorants stood motionless, except for one dark shape that took off and flew away, low down on the water. I could hear the oystercatchers and the curlews, see the gulls whipping away in the wind and I thought to myself:

This is autumn and it is utterly beautiful!

The red leaves of the brambles, the hawthorn berries, even the blackened rosehips beside the path. The slow, slightly lonely joy of walking through the puddles, knowing the family are warm and cosy at home, now that we have turned the heating on for winter.

I had been thinking, early this morning after Dash had settled last night. At first, as may be common with autumn and the passing of the years, I felt regret. I could not name it properly and neither could I name the same contradictory joy within the regret. I was angry with myself, asking how I could have allowed myself to grow so unfit, so that my breath wheezes even when I sit down and I pant when I walk to the top of the stairs. I look at my body and ask how I managed to let my stomach swell so much with so much food, that it is easier to let my shirt hang loose than try to tuck it in under the bulge of it. I worried about the gallons and gallons of whisky I have drunk in recent years, so much whisky that even my skin reeks of it in the morning.

I pondered and felt talons of something unnameable clutching at my spirit and my joy. I cannot name it because I am not sure what it is. Sometimes I think that in trying to come to terms with death, I have let myself bid farewell to life. Increasingly, I dream of oblivion where there is nothing and I am at peace from the pain of my thoughts. Increasingly, I realise that even if I leave a legacy in policy or in words or even in love, it will be even more momentary and transient than life and increasingly, I realise that humanity itself is just a frantic flash of the smallest instant of the smallest instant.

I thought for a time that this was a reckoning and the coming of acceptance but now I fear that I have been saying goodbye too early, getting used to finality before I have even begun.

I fear that the hooks of the past, the memories I hesitate to have faith in have taken their lazy hold of my flesh. I fear that the medication or the illness or whatever it is has finally taken the most savage reckoning of me with my inability to live, to feel joy and lightness.

I woke with that. I woke with that but also with the glimmer of something brighter in my mind. And when I found myself splashing through the puddles at Ardmore, I realised that I do not need to bid farewell and that there is the chance of something bright and that there always was.

How to tell? How to describe my slow smile when, yesterday, Wendy got me to practice smiling and told me that she thought I had never exercised my smiling muscles because all I could do was grimace in a faint parody of joy. How to talk about opening the door to Charlotte's room where she and Orlaith were painting the most beautiful pictures while the rabbits stared in curiosity from behind their mesh curtains? Or this morning, drinking coffee, me sat in my chair, Wendy sitting up in the sofa bed, Dash on his back with his paws dangling in the air above his face. The smell just now of a Halloween cake baking downstairs. The last dramatic, turbulent, traumatic six years of living which still contain joy despite it all. The geese in the fields, the children chattering and scowling. Wendy laughing, being rude, being loving and resolutely untidy; holding the family on a raft of wonder and periodically wondering why she sometimes gets so tired, only to say, "Ah! That is the reason!"

I seek to tear those talons I mentioned earlier, that distort my memory, my zest. I want to celebrate my astonishment that for nearly a decade now I have been in the sort of relationship I would never ever have dared dream was possible for me.

And for once I will celebrate the small steps I am taking to learn to stop imposing darkness on my thoughts. The delighted recognition I have had recently that I am no longer hazy with whisky by nine at night and that I wake after a deep sleep and can face breakfast now with hints of zest and brightness in my mind.

My autumn wish? Such a subtle one. All I need to do is blink to make it true. Learning that, though I pant at the top of the stairs, even though I snore so loudly I have to sleep alone, there are shreds of delight on even the dullest day and that when it is sunny, which it often is, I wake, finding the dandelion blossom is still drifting in the wind, ready to drop with a soft greeting on your shoulder, saying,

"I am still here and I still smile and I still love, despite my lack of practice at it. Despite my fear that I will never get it right!"

Wendy is away out with her friends, all loaded up with cake for their Saturday bake-off. I think she will have fun. She has got dressed up, put on her make up and her jewellery and her cakes taste delicious. I tried one of the failures just a few moments ago!

Earlier, I was at Jean's Bothy for the photography. We did a lot of wittering and I really can't quite remember what it was that we wittered about now, but it drifted in bright sparks, in a lazy, loving way, while we took Christmas postcard themed photos. After that I walked Dash; the water was high, breaking over the rocks and into the rockpools on the point. The sky at this time of the year is often dramatic; in one direction, dark clouds and a silver sea streaked by a seemingly dark sun and in the other, blueness and green fields and little white horses on the water of the bay. Dash was very interested in the sheep. I wonder what he would do if he was in the field and off the lead? I think it might be a disaster!

This month is slightly chaotic and confusing. I can hardly remember much of it at all. I remember, a few days ago I got my jag. My muscles twitched involuntarily, which is always a weird feeling, and my CPN said she would talk to my doctor about counselling for the things in the past that seem to bother and hurt me when they come to life nowadays and catch me unawares. I am pleased about that but not at all certain that there really was a past to be sad about.

Juliet has got me booked up for another perinatal mental health talk and I am not sure whether to do my usual speech or use my creative writing piece on failed fatherhood. I am inclined to the latter, but still cannot decide on its quality!

I got a cheque in for my book week event with Dumbarton area council on alcohol this morning which was very quick indeed. I so wish I could do these events for work instead of the routine of daily work. I sometimes come to life on such occasions, it may all be performance and exhausting, but it can feel exhilarating too.

You know, I don't want to say much to you, whoever you are, this month. I have worked very, very hard. I have been chairing international meeting after international meeting on involuntary treatment and though I say it myself, I think I have done fairly well at it, but I am so crammed full of information that I can hardly think. I am pleased, though, that the more I test what I think we need to do, the more people agree with me. That is a good feeling.

I have worked hard at the Commission too, and had some good conversations, finished some reports. When I reached Friday evening, yesterday, I just slumped on the couch once the children were gone, could hardly keep my eyes open. I don't remember much of what we did. I cuddled up on the couch with Wendy, with Dash joining us at odd moments when he wanted a cuddle.

It is now some weeks since I started drinking only at 9 p.m. on weekdays and that has been so good. It feels strange to say I feel so much more alert because at the moment I am looking forward to when I can give up on this section of writing with a degree of grace and cuddle into my bed and listen to the radio while Dash sleeps at my feet.

The weekends have been busy, the weekdays have been busy and just for the moment I want time to do nothing, achieve nothing. It is strange that it is now over two years since Dad died. I haven't thought of him much since we spread his ashes and when I have, it has been with glimpses of affection instead of grief or unnecessary resentment. I would love to talk to him just now, just to pass the time and let him know what we are all up to. That would be good but I always have my dreams for that if it becomes necessary.

We held our photography exhibition at Jean's Bothy; that was such a lovely day. After the evening of giggling and helping hang the photos, we had a launch event. All of us in the garden with the gazebo. A famous photographer saying stuff, Kath saying stuff, people like me and Janet grinning and feeling both very excited and nervous. We had the shadow minister for health there and our local MP, Brendan O' Hara. He was so lovely and so kind to wee Charlotte. It made me very happy. I got it all wrong, though. I knew I recognised him and for some reason thought he was the mental health team leader who sometimes gives me my jag and talked to him as such and told people like Janet that that was who he was, only to find out, just as he was leaving, that he was our MP! We sold some of the photos and one of mine is being used in a magazine. That feels pretty good.

2019—NOVEMBER—ALAN—MOONLIT DARKNESS WITH WISPY CLOUDS

Yesterday, I had a day in Oban; mainly driving and talking, with the odd visit to a charity shop thrown in.

This is a short, short story. Charlotte went to school fine, all cheery, in fact, with her packed lunch and books. James was cheery too, until, at the school gates, a fellow pupil started asking him about Pokemon. His acute embarrassment at having to interact in front of his family was almost glorious to behold! He ignored the wee boy and shuffled into the playground with his head down and his steps all jerky. Dash the dog was delighted, as this morning was doggy day care day. As soon as he saw Mike coming up the path his whole body started waggling with excitement.

Wendy sat in the car at the station until the last moment (as usual) and dashed out the car with the usual, "Oh fuck!" when the train arrived.

And I set off for Oban. The car was covered in frost in the morning and my coat was smeared with a white haze of ice that had fallen from the window scraper.

It was a great day for driving – some clouds but a lot of sun. The mountains covered in snow but the roads dry enough that the windows didn't get dotted with crud.

On the way to Loch Lomond a pheasant clattered out of the hedge, missing the car by inches. Past Tarbert, I looked across the loch at the youth hostel and remembered that time, all those years ago, when we walked the West Highland Way.

And there was no music because there seems to be no radio signal for most of Argyll once you leave the coast.

I loved when I got to Loch Awe and there were small islands scattered over it, looking half sunken, and I loved when I got to Connell and under the bridge you can see the swirling rapids of the tide; the hump of the wave of water which you would surely drown in.

And once I was in Oban, finding the different addresses I needed to go to, I loved the click of my shoes on the concrete, somehow there is something satisfying about that solid contact. And it was good to stare out at the islands and the fishing boats and the ferries; the seaweed all along the foreshore.

Hope Kitchen was fab, the soup lovely, thick and potatoey and full of carrots and the people were lovely too. Oban FM was great too. I wittered for an hour, felt not only brilliant, but welcomed by everyone.

But the bit I remember most was driving back home in the dark. There was such a bright full moon and atmospheric clouds. Sometimes I would be driving towards the V of a dark glen and that gap would be filled with a smoky yellowy brightness and the darkness of forest. Sometimes I would come to the top of a hill and I would see the soft glow, the sky and the bright round moon. Wonderful! At other times, driving by the still lochs, the water would glow and shimmer in this quiet, ethereal, awe-inspiring way; making me want to stop and sit and just stare at the moonglow.

Finally, after I had picked Wendy up, I went to bed. We had talked, or rather Wendy had talked. I had just been too tired to concentrate on her words. I left as soon as I could, with a brief kiss, and then, snuggled in bed, which was cold because of the nighttime frost, I realised that I have been getting this all wrong.

I am grieving but at the same time I am not. I do not think I have any right to grieve. I feel guilty that sometimes I can sense an undertone of being upset. Everyone is so busy getting on with life. Even Mum, who is not sleeping, is busy doing the life bit, and so am I. I am working. When I look at my diary, I see I have filled it for weeks ahead and it feels like a blow to my stomach because I do not know if I can face all that intensity, that focus, that enthusiasm. I don't want to sit and mourn, as in remember Dad, or cry, but I do want to curl up and walk the dog and stare into space and just rummage around in me for some sense of connection so that I can talk with Wendy and the children, without trying to do so through a layer of wool.

I feel so terribly remote. I would like to be walking up a glen with that moon on the path and in the trees, bundled up in warm clothing, just walking into the sadness.

I would like to be drunk; I would like to be asleep. I would both love to feel and yearn never to feel again.

I contemplated texting Wendy that I had got this dead dad stuff so wrong, but I didn't. I fell asleep and woke to find Dash the dog wriggling around to get comfortable on the bed beside me. In the end, he lay his head on my hips and fell asleep before getting up later to find a different sleeping place.

I woke at two a.m. and stayed awake till five a.m., not thinking anything much, just being awake and finding the radio annoying.

Wendy, as usual, saw I was not quite right in the morning, dragged my story out of me, talked of all sorts to do with grief and then said that it would have been her dad's birthday today. It was good to talk, a relief, but I wish I could have been more helpful over her memories of her dad.

Now I am on the train home, ripping through the freezing fog, the white, frost-laden fields. I wish the train was warmer. I want to work and I want to walk and I want to do nothing and I suspect I will do nothing, not in the way where you breath a sigh of indulgence and gratification but where, after a while, you shift around, fidget at the waste you are making of these dull hours.

I must look out for that moon again tonight, I must learn how to speak and I must learn just why I think I have no right to grieve for my own father.

FROST, POKEMON AND A WILD DOG

I woke to a blue, blue sky; not so cold as usual but still frosty. Well, when I say woke, I had actually woken up at about five thirty and listened to the radio in the dark, radioing away about Brexit and elections and just as it was last night, my soul was dull. I had that ache of emptiness, of not feeling or wanting or anything, really.

It has been a hard, hard week. There have been moments which were wonderful, but when I pause, I just feel like staring and curling up and sleeping and not being here at all. I am still caught on that book I have read that says that the effects of medication are to create that very slowness and bluntness, that lack of feeling I have. I had been assuming that this was what depression was or maybe negative symptoms, but to realise it could also be the effect of the drugs I have been on for the last thirty years, that brought me up short.

My strongest yearning is to find those times when my heart is light and I can giggle; when thoughts dart everywhere in my head and I have words ready to scatter all around me and I am able to laugh and just bounce a bit. That wonderful joy of being alive. It is so rare for me, even more so at the moment. Imagine if I could find that? If I could regain energy and joy and vigour! What would I do for that? That wonderful dream, that wonderful possibility?

I had to choose whether or not to take my medication voluntarily yesterday. Apparently my T3 has expired and Dr Felix asked what I would like – voluntary medication or a DMP. I think he would like me to just agree, and yet I cannot. So at some point, a designated medical practitioner, employed by the very organisation that employs me will come to assess me to see if they should insist on the medication.

This time I am maybe more determined to resist it and yet, when I wittered about it on Twitter and Wendy saw my wittering and dismay, she brought me back; reminded me that this slow whatever it is, is also a symptom of schizophrenia. Just as it is an effect of the drugs and that stopping the drugs would be no guarantee of a change in me, would send me back to the devils and things, which would be even worse.

In the mood I am in at the moment, it just made me so, so, terribly sad, as if there is no escape. That this experience is permanent. That there is no prospect of hope. I do not think I can come to terms with this reality.

I go to sleep as soon as I can nowadays, keep an eye out for the excuse that means that I can reasonably retreat to my bed without offending Wendy, and there I feel some safety. I feel glad when Dash wakes me when he wriggles on the bed in the middle of the night, glad when it is two in the morning and I know I can lie alone and silent and not thinking, just lying there on my own, staring into the darkness.

And I do feel so guilty that I am somehow not coping. It seems to me that I do not have any right at all to be sad, that I should be getting on with life. At the same time it also feels like I am being self indulgent, wallowing in a way no one else is. I feel guilty because I do not feel sad about Dad. I do not think of him much at all but I feel pale and insubstantial. I feel delicate, as though I might need to rush out of a work meeting, give up work, argue at work. Wendy says I was his son, that it is just weeks since he died, but it doesn't seem to me that I have any right at all to be so seemingly pathetic about all this. I do not believe I should be upset. I do not feel I am allowed to be upset, and in some ways I am not. Except I do not feel anymore at all and I have lost the little energy I used to have.

And yet, when I got up this morning, I said, 'Good morning, beautiful!' in my text to Wendy, to let her know the coffee was on. Because she is beautiful and I am not paying her attention in the way that I should. My heart lifted slightly when she came down, all tousled. Out of the window we could see this blue, cloudless sky.

Wendy keeps an eye on me all the time at the moment, worries that I am not in as good a place as I say I am. I am lucky in this, so lucky. Last night Charlotte hugged and hugged me before she went to bed and Wendy talked, and her voice and her reason soothed, but still I would so much love to sleep and sleep and sleep.

STRETCHING FOR THE PLEASURE OF IT

Dash is taking up too much of the downie. It is so cold today and I have not put the heating on, so the bits of me that are in the air are shrinking a bit.

I think today is the very first day in which I have felt normal. I am not exhausted, I am not blank with that lack of being. I am not thinking of Dad and I am not thinking I have no right to grieve.

I have just been busy. I forgot how good it could be to be busy, how much it can take you away from your thoughts; that gape of not feeling, not connecting.

I can't remember breakfast except that, unusually for her, Wendy had Marmite on her toast. These little things that we notice! I remember we grumbled about the politics on the telly. I know that yet again we watched the BBC London channel because the Freeview box Wendy got from the charity shop is tuned to English TV channels and I know I contemplated finding out which channel is Scotland so we could just turn to that each morning but I didn't, as usual. I often think of doing that but never do.

We were up earlier than we needed as we thought Tom would drop the children off when he came to pick up their school bags but he was too late for that, so I emptied the dishwasher, put a wash on, put the clothes on to dry. And then I was busy scraping the ice off the car. I used the ice defroster, feeling guilty, as I am sure it is very un-eco. I realised that our white car is now nearly a brown car and then we were at the station, waiting for the late train to arrive.

After dropping Wendy off, I went on my usual trip to Ardmore with Dash the dog. I so love this walk, never get bored of it. Last night I even drove down to it on my way back from work to take photos as it looked breathtaking in the setting sun with the cloudless sky. Stunning.

Today there was a band of fog lying over the hills near Dunoon, where my sister Juliet lives, and nearer to us, tendrils of mist rising from the still water of the Clyde and a morning sun making everything bright. The sun was hot enough that I did not need gloves, the air cold enough that ice crystals covered the grass and the leaves. The puddles were thickly frozen; my breath filling the air with steam. And Dash, very happy, and now that we have gone back to the cheese treats, much better behaved. He had a lovely time rushing backwards and forwards and dashing up to me when I offered cheese when I called him, sometimes literally skidding to a halt when he reached me.

I did not think much on my walk; just stared at the white frozen ground, my favorite tree in the field with the sheep, the sun on the water, that bank of cloud, that bright sky above it.

Then we were driving into the bright, dazzling sun for bin bags in Dumbarton, going to the car wash and at last being able to see out the windows without a veil of dirt obscuring our vision. Back home, packing bag after bag of the clothes Wendy has put out for the charity shops, only just fitting them into the car.

And the busyness has kept me more or less bright.

My mum is busy being invited places nowadays, but I have no idea how she is doing; she is still not sleeping, I know that much. Still having hassle over names and bills and things like this.

I can still remember those seals from Saturday, the two basking on a rock by the water's edge. The other one that swam up to them and hoiked itself out the water to lie beside them. We watched them for ages. I think the bit I liked best was when they arched their backs, raising their flippers way into the air. It looked like such a luxurious response to the day.

I think I would like to do that. It seems so long since I have stretched with pleasure, just stretched and grinned and wondered what to do with the day. I would like to do that and to turn round and laugh with Wendy. I do laugh, but I would like to laugh as if I hadn't a worry in the world.

2021—NOVEMBER—MENTAL HEALTH AND ME— GEILSTON: A PLACE OF HEALING, LAUGHTER AND BIRDSONG

It must be six years ago that we took wee James home from the ICU in the Sick Kids in Glasgow. I remember those days vividly: Wendy's description of the relatives room, the beeping machines, James when he came out of his induced coma, asking for a blueberry muffin. Me, walking the streets while waiting for Wendy, hoping my new family would survive and then, just a couple of days after that muffin, under that huge tree in the walled garden in the bright blue of summer. James and Charlotte, cuddling and dancing and tottering on the grass by the tree. Us. Grinning, laughing, the horror of the last few days not exactly fading but slipping aside for a moment.

Geilston was the perfect setting for the start of James's recovery. The haze of the trees, with green grass and flowers and birdsong. A picnic, a rug; the delight of life continuing, when for a while it had hung in the balance with nurses studying machines, parents caught on the dread of the worst ever news and me, the new member of the family; giving the lifts, tidying the house, making meals until we allowed ourselves to smile and Wendy started her constant journeys upstairs to check her now healthy son was still breathing while he slept.

Geilston has been, until recently, the place we love to go to. James's favourite place. The place we walk by the burn, play Pooh Sticks with pine cones on one of the little bridges. We find fairies here, and toadstools. We have sat under the pergola for picnics and we have swung from rhododendron bushes. We have looked at swathes of daffodils, loved the bluebells. We have sat on the carved mushrooms at the play bit where the children climb on the netting. I have lost to both James and Charlotte at the tennis and tried to pretend I meant to. The children have chased us up and down the flowery maze until we are breathless. James has burst into tears when our hide and seek was too good, up at the white bench where the orchard starts.

The children have peered at the plants, the pumpkins. James has led us on bizarre journeys, on Easter Egg hunts with his map held upside down in front of his face, sure he knows the way, looking forward to his 'free' chocolate.

We have sat on the benches at the entrance, talking to the staff, drinking our drinks and eating our snacks, wondering which of the vegetables to buy from the stand beside us.

It is a lovely, lovely place to sit and walk and ponder and wonder and also a lovely place where children shriek with laughter and have wondrous mini adventures.

Of course, it is not just a place for children, it is a place for everyone.

I sometimes go there to sit on a bench to write on my laptop; to rest and muse with the maze of the green light, the slight sound of the trickle of the water.

I have a lovely life but can struggle to connect to the world and the people around me. My family are without a shadow of doubt the people that give me the wonderful life I have. The NHS most probably keeps me functioning but one of the things that really keeps me alive and filled with the pleasure that I live where I do, is the wonder of the fresh air and the natural world.

I find walking can calm my thoughts, the motion of my body soothes my muscles, reduces the chatter of thoughts I do not want to have. Sitting beside a peat-dark river, the water sliding softly past, can lull me into a softness. Looking at the beauty of flowers and the motion of the birds inspires me. Walking in the soft mistiness of the trees makes my breath soft and happy. I once wrote an article saying that nature is our Natural Health Service and for me, at least, that is true.

It may be taking Dash the dog for walks at Ardmore but it is also ambling among flowers in places like Geilston; looking at the trees heavy with blossom; looking at the old house and saying to Wendy, "Imagine if that was renovated? If people could come here to write, sing, dance or draw or just sit. Imagine if this was a place where I could just pause to watch the sunset or a place where we could listen to music or cook a meal?"

We used to imagine winning the lottery and buying Geilston for the people of Cardross but wanted to be able to live there too! But that was our idle imagination. Now I hear, one day, it may be a place where activities like that happen because of the efforts of people who, unlike us, acted on their dreams to keep it open.

For me, there is something wonderful about seeing vegetables growing, apples ripening. To walk in no particular direction between the trees, ending up in the walled garden.

Imagine if this were a place we could all go to? To find peace and refuge and the delight in knowing we can relax with the wonder of the green grass, the bright flowers, so many butterflies in summer; the welcome of the staff when we walk into the vegetable garden.

This place is a place that gives me room to breathe and smile; room to laugh and dare to roll down the hill with the children in the height of summer. When being dizzy and filled with the scent of soil and vegetation makes me understand how precious the world really is when sometimes I struggle to realise this.

December

2021—DECEMBER—WENDY—A NON LOVE LETTER TO FINISH UP WITH

When I walked into the room today, Wendy and the children were in hysterics, having improvised a theatre company out of James's Fortnite characters that he got for Christmas. Wendy was centre stage and, with many weird voices, they were mapping out the life of the greeny-grey thing with a big head. I think they had decided he needed bullied because they hated him and had taken him to the top of a large bridge where they were planning his murder!

Later, when we were lying on our respective couches among the detritus of Christmas, we decided doing things like this can be good and healthy. For children as well behaved as Charlotte and James, make believe and saying things you know you shouldn't say, and which should never happen, is a great, great liberation from the puritanism we seem to be stuck with where we, especially children, are so frightened of saying or thinking the wrong thing that we even censor our own thoughts. Sometimes we need the freedom to express ourselves in all the worst ways, in the safety of our families where we will not cause harm or we become frightened robots, hasty to judge and censor anything that deviates from convention. Cultivating the ability to shock and think in ways that are inexcusable? There can be something in that sometimes; where you just stop behaving and find freedom in the unacceptable.

I was tumbling today. Relieved to get out with Dash the dog and yet angry with Wendy for not coming with me. As I walked the path, I grumped about her, built up a huge raft of resentment. Of course, all the usual things: about not being praised or admired or adored every time I walk into a room. An accumulation of a year of close company where we cannot be as close and free and spontaneous as we wish, either because we need space, Wendy is in pain from her endometriosis, the children are sharing her bed or snuggling in between us, or we are still winding down from Zoom or Teams or the washing needs folded, the shopping done, tea cooked; the things that make it hard just to relax with each other.

That accumulation of months of stress and the strain of trying to be pleasant and the tension of not being free with the joy we know we have in each other's company. I had a list of things I imagined I would confront Wendy with when I returned home, knowing full well I wouldn't.

Sitting in the oversized armchair, I watched the last of the very first version of *A Star is Born*, which Wendy was absorbed in and moved by. At the end she turned to me and fell into animated conversation, but first she said she knew I wanted us to tidy the house but she needed a few hours not doing anything responsible, that she was getting irritable and angry at minor things.

She said that now the children were away with their dad, her mum happy with Christmas, her staff on holiday, she needed time not to feel or be responsible for anything, not even for me.

I liked that and that is why this final section is no romantic journey among the clouds and dandelion parachutes. While I made her tea and poached eggs on toast, we talked about this and that, mainly about Judy Garland who seems to have had the most horrendous life and been abused by the most horrendous people.

Life feels very responsible now. Covid, work, children, age and health have stolen a lot of my laughter and joy from me and I fear that Wendy's spontaneity and everyday joy in life is sometimes severely put to the test. Sometimes when you are exhausted, it is impossible to relax, to twirl round the kitchen in hugs and kisses or to spend an evening chatting and laughing.

The last few weeks, work has been so intense and feels so important. This carries its own pressure, especially when trying to navigate amongst opposing views and feeling very, very alone. Having my mum to visit was a joy but it was hard to turn the off switch. The excitement of Christmas and presents and panto and so on, wonderful, but again, no time. No smooth expanse of hours where we do nothing except wash away the tension of the last few months and learn not to perform or please and instead, snuggle up to caress and giggle but mainly sleep.

I did think our head in the clouds, parachute-kissed, blue sky existence would carry on and on and on for ever and ever with no effort which, finally I realise, is slightly naïve. It doesn't lessen our love for each other but it has been tempered by responsibility, which is something I have an uneasy relationship with.

We often have conversations about how the debate and discussion of feminism seems to have got it all wrong; that the issues like sharing equally in the domestic tasks are really very out of date when what needs to be talked about is the pressure to nurture and look after and cheer up and create laughter and conversation. That this seems to still be very much the realm of women or, at least, women in families.

How can I take Wendy's hand and take her to the side of a stream to cuddle up together, or snuggle up on the couch, or whisper sweet nothings to her at night while we watch some rom com when what she most needs is a rare moment of space for herself? A chance not to be making anyone else feel good about themselves or creating a happy atmosphere; just the chance to zone out and watch crap on telly and eat chocolate and crisps?

It is the time of resolutions. While we were watching *A Star is Born*, Wendy told me that one of the most moving scenes was when Judy Garland said, "Sometimes love is not enough," as her husband became more and more ill from the alcohol he consumed.

I am slowly beginning to drink less but my inner landscape is still one filled with demons and darkness and torment. I imagine Wendy might ask herself the same thing. Why? When she pours love into my life every day, do I still feel as bad as I possibly can about myself? Why is this schizophrenia stuff still thundering away? It must be exhausting.

Many years ago she said she was very happy to look after family, look after everything but needed to know that she was also supported and could know she was safe in another person's love. Such an important lesson for me. I fear she has found out that, far from being the person who keeps her safe, I have slowly turned into another family member needing reassured; only snuggled up to after the children are done, the rabbits put to bed, the dog's prescription dealt with.

My resolution is to go back to the love letters she makes faces at; to carry on cleaning the house and walking the dog, but to find those moments when she can just *stop* without thinking about the next time she needs to deal with whoever it is's anxiety over whatever it is. To do the petals in warm bath thing but also to take some of the responsibility I so easily discard when someone else can take it for me.

I will return to my love letters soon, but they will be based on real events where we have the time to walk hand in hand being silly; go back to row that rowing boat on the loch like we did in the summer; waking up in the morning with no list getting prepared in my head for what we need to do that day to make it a good one. Just the knowledge that it already is.

Knowing that the next few days, while the children are away, we will be able to sleep as long as we want, do what we want, find moments of space and togetherness while letting the pressure of expectation drift into the peace of acceptance and companionship and small reminders of why we love each other.

2021—DECEMBER—MY JOURNAL

My year is coming to an end and I have very mixed feelings indeed about it. The last few days have been both good and bad. It's Christmas Eve. I woke up late, listened to *Desert Island Discs* from bed, made the family scrambled eggs for breakfast, all the things I like to do and yet I feel flat, maybe worse than flat. I cannot see any lightness in me and I know it is irritating my family.

My mum came up from England. That was wonderful, but I had few words and left her and Wendy talking each evening so I could go to bed and sleep. My dreams have been totally bizarre: finding myself in Africa in the fifties, or in an airship sometime in the future, having to fill in satisfaction and wellbeing surveys. I wish I would laugh at it all.

I got my booster very early on via work and that feels good; Wendy got hers as soon as she was entitled to. We are not socialising, though tomorrow we go across town for a Christmas meal with Peter, Sharon, Clare, David and assorted children. I have bought Wendy her presents and I think she will like them. I managed OK with her birthday presents too and she loves the robot hoover, though is that really a present?

I don't know what it is but I am utterly exhausted and all I want to do is to curl up in bed and sleep.

If my real life had been following a story as it should be, I know what I would be doing. Dad would be dead and loved and I would be free from him in my dreams. But I was struck by how Mum said one evening, when she was up here, that he was, for much of his life, an incredibly difficult man, and my heart gave a little leap, a, 'Yes, he was, wasn't he!' A temptation to say, "I was hurt by him a bit too much for my own good," and then I remembered Mum's heartrending sentence in her letter of 'I miss him so much.'

In real life there are no neat endings and my dad will resist being packaged up and sorted tidily away as I seem to wish to do. Because in the next sentence my mum said that he was a lovely man underneath it all and so he was. I just wish I had been able to connect with his loveliness more. I wish the distance I have put between myself and the world was not there so I could laugh freely, so I could have known how to have the sort of conversations he slipped into so easily with Wendy. I wish, in his later years, when we knew we loved each other after all, we could have avoided the middle class understated way in which we expressed our love. So! I have not sorted out my feelings or even my grief for Dad, as is almost a requirement for a book about death and loss, but I am not necessarily sure that it bothers me. After all, why would I want to come to resolutions and closure and the categorisation of complex feelings? No. Let them remain complex, let me continue to meet him in my sleep and remember him smiling from his so deeply tanned face in the summer time, with his book, the remains of lunch on the table and his beer just finished. I would like that he is no problem to be solved and no trauma to be got over with. He's my dad. Like me, he made many mistakes, like everyone, he made many mistakes, but he was my dad and he helped make me, gave me a rich and fascinating life to inhabit.

Covid isn't over. Of course it isn't! We are hardly likely to march into a bright dawn where health becomes a given once again because it never was in the first place. I can easily imagine being one of the last people to actually die from it now it seems to be less severe as, though I hate to say it, I am terribly, terribly unfit at the moment. Overweight, not liking the steps to the top of the house. Grumping when Wendy and my mum say I should see the doctor about my wheezy chest.

My mental health? I had thought I would be on a journey to something new but I am not. I am not as utterly convinced just now that I am bringing the world to an end, but each new typhoon, flood and famine still makes me pretty certain. I am just not too sure now what I should do about it. I do nowadays, occasionally, after I say, "I want to die," reply to myself in a very awkward and self conscious way, telling myself that I don't want to die after all. And in some ways I don't. I will never be able to convey to you how bewilderingly fortunate I have been to find

Wendy in my life and to have the children, Dash, the rabbits, or even, just now, the sound of geese flying overhead. They make schizophrenia, or whatever it is, something less horrific. So much of my life is filled with laughter and my glumness and distance seems for some impossible reason to be accepted as just a part of who I am.

I met my MHO recently and she smilingly said, "We must be reaching the time of year for your tribunal," which we are, and as usual it terrifies me, whatever the outcome. As usual, I will say I want talking treatments and as usual, they will say they will look into it. Maybe it will even become a recorded matter and as usual, after a few months they will stop even talking about providing it.

Someone at work keeps on saying how people with a mental illness need to take responsibility for themselves as part of their recovery journey and I can't describe how irritated that makes me and how even more irritated I am that some of us sign up to such things. If I acted responsibly, I would walk in front of the Caledonia Sleeper tonight. That might delay the end of the world a little, remove one of the elements of negativity that are destroying the world. If I was responsible, I would leave the Scott Review as I am sure that I am influencing it in some way to the detriment of the community I feel I belong to. In many ways I feel I have been far too responsible all my life. I have worked so hard at something that anyone with any sense would know will never have a good outcome. The responsible and insightful action would have been to have known the pressure it put me and my family under and my current family and circle of friends. If, when I had first cracked up properly, all those years ago, when my son was born, I had accepted the advice of those around me and claimed disability benefits, stopped working so hard, maybe I would have learnt to live a warmer, kinder life. Maybe I would still see my son, maybe my wife would not have become so bitter and done the things she did.

It is a little silly, reflecting on the might-have-been, and a little silly for me to contemplate stopping work as I know I won't and would only do what I do now voluntarily, if I did. But it is a relief to finally know that I edge closer and closer to the love of family and life and more and more want to see work as the bit that allows the best bits to happen.

Threaded in some of my thoughts these last few months have been the so, so fashionable thoughts of the past and trauma. Such an important thing for so many people but so easy for someone like me to fall into and lose myself in.

The policeman phoned me to say that that teacher is finally being charged and unless he pleads guilty, I will have to appear in court. He also said that the teacher is also being charged with indecent assault against me which I wasn't prepared for. It made me irritable and not the best person to work with for some days. Is any of it trauma? I hate that memories flood me, but know my life was mainly one of privilege and had considerable laughter in it.

Yes. School was bad, being sent away from home was bad and confusing, moving house all the time was awful, but I remember Wendy talking about her own childhood and saying that she always knew she was loved and that was the most important thing.

Much as I labour the point, that I felt I was sent away because I was not loved, I have always, despite my best efforts, known how much love there always was in my family.

I witness people devastated by trauma so often, I have had the good fortune to have only glimpsed some of the harsher aspects of life and to have friends and family who are able to put up with me when I get maudlin, able to accept me as me, which is so good.

I did fail though, sometime at the beginning of this. I wanted to live as though I had no illness, as though I was free of the weight of it all. Now I see that written down baldly, it doesn't make sense, but then neither does my assertion that I have no illness and am instead a devil rest easy with my acceptance that I might have schizophrenia. Neither does my easy assumption that I see myself in a very, very poor light and assume everyone else does, when just today Wendy was trying to help me see that the negatives we all have are tiny in the grand scheme of things, but it determines how I view myself and how I describe myself. I wanted to be free of the distance between me and the world. I have this memory that once I saw and felt the world in colour and I can almost remember such times and yet the decades and decades of being remote from feeling and vibrance and just being alive, it wears me down. Sometimes I feel so alien and such a poor example of humanity. Over this year some people have continued to tell me that they see me as autistic. I do wonder at that. I certainly don't 'get' people and can be bewildered when I get into trouble with the things I say but had no idea were offensive.

Where am I in my mental health journey? I am happier. I would say I sometimes doubt I am all that is evil, or at least doubt it more than I did, but after last night's dream where I found myself in various versions of hell and woke to spend the rest of the night realising just how much damage I cause and how important it is that I deal with my reality, I find myself lost. But then, like Sandy and my dad said, 'It is what it is,' however trite a phrase that might be.

I am dreading Christmas tomorrow. The morning with the children will be good but later: me, Dash, Wendy's mum, the chihuahua? What a combination! My temptation will be to drink too much, say nothing and hope everyone wants to go to bed early; strange how confusing even the loveliest of families can be and my apprehension when I know really it will be lovely.

I call myself a writer but I don't know even its basic rules. I imagine that out of a story comes a crisis and a resolution, the suspense ends and we all go our various, slightly more fulfilled ways. It is a nice thing to witness, this neat and optimistic ending where the baddies are packed off and the lovers reconciled. I still have my schizophrenia, there were no baddies really, not really much of a tragedy. Two fairly elderly men died and we were all affected by both their deaths and their dying, and in different ways still are. I started the year in love with Wendy and finish the year in love with her and I am delighted by that. She is still as wild and crude and funny as ever. The children are living their story. It is an exciting one, of which I will only witness a little, but I love being at its beginning. My son? Some tiny movement there; I heard in a sparse but so welcome sentence that he now lives in Kyrgyzstan and is content and safe. In my world that is gift enough. It kept me smiling for days. Imagine if one day I heard from him once more? Imagine if one impossible day I could actually meet him again!

My work? To have a resolution to a job like mine would be to wake up to the press in the morning saying that world peace had broken out and we have all learnt how to love and be kind to each other and that distress and despair is a thing of the past. Not really going to happen!

I think, as usual, my resolution to this story or year is that there are no resolutions. I haven't a clue what will happen in the future. Dash will still cuddle up in the evening and want his walks. James will play his computer games, Charlotte will do something arty and grow even more mature with her emotions than she already is. I will still dream of being a successful writer whilst at the same time knowing that if I ever became publicly successful at anything, I would hate it. Wendy will remind me that when I die I will not lie there and say how good I was at my job, instead I will remember people that I love or things like the joy of eating a family picnic while the world does all the world things it has always done and which I have no chance of or need to understand. Wendy, what will she get up to? She will make fun of life and she will laugh about life and she will love and treasure, she will continue to be a wonderful worker, a person curious about the world and so, so clever. She says she has decided that she will spend the rest of her life with me, however irritating I get. She will go on another diet after Christmas because however silly that is, that is what people do. I would love to have the kindness she doesn't know how to set aside, even when she hates the world!

My coffee has gone cold, Wendy is having a shower, the telly is noisy in the other room and after lying down on the sofa bed to write this, I feel pretty good. Maybe I am a bit flat just now, but in half an hour I will be walking Dash by the sea while Wendy and the children visit her mum. We will come home to food and a warm house and might stop off to buy some Ben and Jerry's ice cream before settling down for the rest of Christmas Eve.

My resolution I made in July? No, I didn't achieve it! For so much of my life, my existence lives smothered in cotton wool. Drinking less has helped a bit, taking my antidepressants has helped a bit, but I suppose it is just a part of my existence, this gap between me and the world. I promised to give the family a bit more joy and to take more responsibility and to help Wendy not be in charge of everything. Work is some sort of an excuse for failing at this. It has been incredibly busy and incredibly stressful, the only way I have managed to keep on doing it has been because of the support and help of Simon on the secretariat at the review; he seems to instinctively understand my constant anxiety and self doubt and to put it at ease. I went through a time when I really thought I should resign and give up, but the gentle support of him and some others have helped me realise that although this is a stressful thing we are doing, and incredibly complex, that it is slowly gaining coherence and the possibility that we will all be agreeing in what we say, maybe a bit idealistic but is at least not something I shrink from thinking about anymore. It feels strange how, just a short while ago I was so paranoid and that now I tend to look forward to meetings and papers and reports and all the people involved in this work. I wish I knew them better, but every day there is another scrap of evidence of their kindness and integrity.

The pressure of this work, or my work with the Commission, is not really an excuse however, especially as I also do my writing, especially as I retreat to write this book, do the Instagram posts. It is maybe important for me to recognise that, to see my own uncertainty damages other people too.

We are talking about maybe being able to buy a bigger house next year, if I can sell my own house. It would be lovely to each have a bedroom to sleep in and somewhere to work from. It would be lovely to have most of the mortgage paid off. Sometimes Wendy says that when the review finishes I should not take back my hours, maybe decrease them further. The thought of that has an appeal. I think I could become more supportive and less anxious if I wasn't trying to prove myself through the achievement and activity of work. Maybe I could become, as I promised myself, a better part of the family, more likely to be there for everyone, more likely to find time to make sure Wendy does not have to stay up late to get her own me-time.

In many ways, my all too obvious lesson from this year's puzzling about life and the last six years of love and laughter since moving here is this: I will continue to love the mist on the sea, ice cream, working out the school lunch, cuddling the dog, learning to sleep. Being a part of something I didn't dare dream I could have, learning to love life and the people in my life and maybe even me, and to forgive myself for whatever I need to forgive myself for.

And of course, knowing one day it will all stop and that somehow that might not matter too much, there really is nothing better than talking together over coffee in the morning, death does not have to be terrifying, achievement is suspect, closure a weird thing. I think my main lesson to myself is this: I will never understand myself or the world around me but I do not need to. I will not package my life. Instead, I will look forward to when next I see curlews tumbling in the wind and windsurfers scudding on the water, Wendy making fun of everything, dancing like I will one day!

That December after Dad died, I had planned to write about it. I know I went down to see Mum for her birthday as I was worried about her being alone in the house. Well, I didn't go for her birthday. Instead, I arrived a few days after it but the intention was there.

I thought I would have lots to say about those days so soon after Dad died and so soon in Mum's journey without him but now that I think about it, I cannot remember it at all, or hardly. I have looked up Instagram, where I remark on all these things, and have found out I wasn't on it by then. I have looked up Facebook and found a few sparse photos.

There is one of a huge rain cloud. I remember that walk. We managed to dodge the rainstorms when I thought it would pour on us for certain. That is all I remember; the photograph makes me remember how vivid the sky was, how dark the cloud. It makes me think of the pebbly beach and the wetlands, the old mill ruins. It doesn't remind me of my conversations with my mum.

There is another post where I mention that I am about to take Mum out for her birthday meal, but I don't remember that either.

I have no idea where we went or what we did for those few days. I cannot remember our conversations, what I bought her for her birthday, what the rest of the family was up to.

I have a vague memory that we went to the cinema in Lewes to watch a strange and slightly depressing film and I remember we ate in its restaurant. That we liked the meal very much and that maybe we had got the train there so I could have a drink.

I remember Mum was not sleeping well. That is about all I remember. She could no longer sleep like she used to and before that time, when she used to sleep, she already slept badly and that now she was sleeping even worse than usual. It worried me. I know what a world is like when you cannot sleep and are besieged by thoughts and memories.

I think we would have reassured ourselves, as we had already, that Dad had died so quickly and that it really was the release we were all saying it was. That in some remarkable way, Dad had said goodbye to most of the important people in his life in the months before his final heart attack. That those months had been good ones but that he really was becoming more and more ill and that life for him and Mum had been looking grim indeed.

He stayed in the house and did not have to go into care which he dreaded. We never had to enact his power of attorney, which was just as well, as he refused to give any indication of what his wishes would be if he lost capacity. I remember those frustrating conversations, asking as delicately as I could what he would like to happen when that time came, him saying he would leave all that to our capable hands.

Apart from that, nothing. Mum was probably just starting back with her volunteering with the Samaritans. But otherwise it is all blank.

It seems fitting. I have come to the end of the year, at the beginning of which I was just coming off of sick leave due to some of the grief that I was feeling for my dad. I have written about my coming to terms with it all, if that is what I have been doing. I have met my dad so often in my dreams but now, now it is becoming a story I am not too confident of.

I am not sure how I feel. Part of me is sad that I can now really only visualise my dad's face, nut brown from the sun, with a beer and a book, or that funny attempt we made at a barbecue, the last time we saw him. How he got the barbecue out, our mutual congratulations and finally, the tiny pile of coals on which we could not cook anything which made for an evening of giggles.

I feel as though I am deserting him but maybe this is what we need to do; to leave our loved ones in peace from the needs of our living demands. To let them fade as we in turn will fade.

It seems a bit to final to say that. So I won't. Instead, when I phone Mum tonight, I will ask her what she remembers of that birthday. We will create a new story of sorts.

2021—DECEMBER—MENTAL HEALTH AND ME— STORYTELLING AS AN AGENT OF CHANGE

Last week I listened to a group from CAPS Independent Advocacy , who I used to work for in Edinburgh, more than quarter of a century ago, telling their stories on Zoom to create change, increase understanding and develop some form of connection. It was wonderful but very alarming to realise that some of the people who had found the courage to speak out weren't even born when I first started working there.

I loved their articulacy; the enthusiasm and the beauty of stories imbued with sadness. I heard about lives that had grown into the most touching and moving stories which could educate and explain and cross bridges.

I always learn something new when I hear someone's story, but this time, far from understanding more about life with a mental illness, I was reminded of the bond of speaking out together; that liberation of knowing you are making a difference and standing alongside your peers. That was wonderful; to find a memory of connection and shared purpose and, of course, that dream of a hope that the future may one day be different.

Storytelling and narrative is often talked about nowadays as a catalyst for change and recovery.

I first told my story publicly, thirty seven years ago in a smoke-filled room in Sheffield, with a group of volunteers and residents of a halfway house for young people. I talked about my stay in one of the old asylums and my subsequent life. Out of the tears and hugs and new stories that accompanied it, came renewed enthusiasm for creating what eventually became McMurphy's, a drop-in centre for young people, run by young people.

It was eight years later when I first started speaking very publicly. It was terrifying! A packed conference in a posh hotel in Edinburgh; me knocking my chair off the back of the stage when I stood up to speak, rushing off when the applause came, to smoke cigarette after cigarette in the hallway before I calmed down and smiled again.

Over the years of telling stories, I saw changes occurring. When I was touring Scotland with the Understanding Psychosis Roadshow, I would get to a certain bit, when I talked about my son, and find my eyes would film over and my voice tremble for a few moments until I was able to carry on speaking in a clearer, more confident manner. People would come up afterwards and congratulate me. Often they were family members who, with tearful voices, told me that I had given them some hope that their child might also have a good life despite having a diagnosis like mine, of schizophrenia.

Slowly, the emotion went and although I was always keyed-up and nervous, I became used to the conference halls; my fear and emotion reduced. I was still always shaky at the end but I began to wonder what to say to people who came up to me. Sometimes I wanted to say that I was just lucky, that there was no reason to believe their son would find the motivation to wander the country or have a family or work just because I had had that good fortune.

By the time I was working in the Highlands with an advocacy group called HUG (Action for Mental Health), storytelling and using our lives was integral to nearly all of what we did.

We used our experiences and our stories to work out, collectively, how change should occur in everything from detention to employment to the environment. The reports we wrote were illustrated with our experiences and, in many cases, services and policy changed, reflecting the voice of our members.

We used our stories to educate the actors and playwrights taking plays around Highland schools. They acted as the bedrock for films and animations that aimed to raise awareness.

Like a minister in a sermon, we would take scraps of our lives and use them to give integrity to our views when in committee meetings, at workshops and when speaking at conferences or at art events.

Finally, and most importantly, we used our stories when trying to educate and increase the awareness of health and social care professionals and the public.

We worked together, and over many years learnt how to craft our stories and give a breadth and depth to them in the training we provided. We would support each other before and afterwards; we trained together, we debriefed together and eagerly looked at the evaluation forms after each event, which showed that testimony, as we called it, was crucial to what we did.

An evaluation of two years of awareness sessions gave scores of 94% excellent and 6% very good for our testimony, carried out with everyone from prison officers to councillors, student nurses to mental health officers.

It was a wonderful and truly exciting way of creating change, and with support and organisation, was usually an enriching experience for our members.

I would like to stop there. To say, "Use our stories. Get us into the open, as happens more and more in so many mediums. Let our stories guide your services!" But when I reflect on my own experience, I have some qualms that might do well to be aired.

My story is crafted. I use different elements to make different points and get across certain messages. I make it interesting, I make it moving but not too moving. I make it graphic but not too graphic. I do not tell people what to think, instead I tend to give a narrative that will let people reach their own conclusions. I have spoken to support workers in Portree in Skye, welfare rights workers in Dingwall. I have spoken at local, regional, national and international events. I have even spoken at the United Nations. I have spoken on film, on telly, on the radio and in the papers, and always I use my story and the stories of others who are happy to for me to use their story. I have written a memoir about my life and received wonderful reviews. I continue to use my story now that I work with the Mental Welfare Commission for Scotland.

I am no longer worried about resurrecting past trauma I might have experienced. I tend to know how to keep my audience safe. I am pretty certain that people won't be bored and fairly sure we will have a good discussion. I know most people will go away with things to think about and reflect on.

What I am worried about is the process of storytelling and of narrative. In the early years, I think telling my story was, in some way, part of the journey of recovery, in that it made sense of my life and took away much of the shame and secrecy that used to surround mental illness.

However, I am hugely grateful that when I was in the Highlands we never dreamed of making our stories the classical recovery story, as in *we got to a better place in our lives* sort of thing. The dangers of such things should be self-evident as, of course, our lives are very rarely rosy and very rarely have wonderful outcomes. What I sometimes worry about for those of us for whom this is almost a career, is the impact of turning our life over and over again into that beautiful creation – a story.

But a story is just that – a story! It has beginnings and endings and usually points and meanings and dramas. Our lives are much more important and vibrant than mere stories. They are not meant to have a plot or a learning point or even a self-imposed direction. I should not start speaking and realise, although I am genuinely talking about my life, I am still only telling a story with a slight scrap of me as a central character who I find distorts my vision of who I really am.

I have created a character that I don't always feel is actually me, with experiences I have, but not all the time, and an identity that does not always feel like my identity. An identity I would sometimes like to leave behind, especially on social media.

There is so much more to me than the story of detention and schizophrenia and isolation and discrimination, or even the story of activism or of recovery or turmoil, oppression or for that matter, liberation!

If I gave an honest and more accurate story I would spent most of my time talking about today's walk in the snow with my partner and our daft dog; the minestrone soup we had for lunch, the emails I answered and the slow breakfast that lazy days off without the children are sometimes composed of. I would not tell a tale that has drama in it and high emotion, that reveals the wonders of the help I get and the pits of when it harms me, in order to make a point and help people learn.

I would not find myself beginning to inhabit that inner thread of illness, casting aside as irrelevant the sound of oystercatchers on the shore, the slow swell of the frozen sea yesterday and the children's red cheeks, in favour of the last time my CPN could not get the injection right and had to go for help to work out what to do while my shirt spotted with blood as I waited.

I worry that when we immerse ourselves in a life-long campaign of activism and speaking out, where our illness and treatment story is central to our identity, that it seeps into our everyday life and we find ourselves lost in a story we have constructed which we do not always fit into and from which we sometimes can't escape.

And yet, these stories, these glimpses into real life are, after all, a sure-fire way of making a difference to the thoughts and attitudes of so many people! I much prefer to learn from real people than PowerPoint slides but I wonder what we do to those like me, who choose to be the story instead of write the slide?

2019—DECEMBER—SANDY—CHRISTMAS

As Christmas drew near, Sandy planned amazing presents for the children.

In the room with the military books, loosely covered in a blanket, was a massive llama-type thing, not as big as the unicorn from last year but nearly as big, far bigger than Charlotte. And in a corner, far posher but far smaller, was the toy sausage dog James had been craving, sausage dogs being his favourite dog and he, still half-convinced he was part dog.

Sandy was determined to give us all a good Christmas meal. We were trying to work out where to go when I found the Queen of the Loch, a pub-type restaurant that took dogs.

It was still a good time then, really. Looking back, I have such mixed feelings. A certainty that Sandy's last months were as good as they could be, but also I remember the tiredness.

That set of Christmas events were lovely. Sandy's last Christmas. I remember the morning. The children were at Tom's for Christmas morning. I think he had forgotten they were coming to us at lunchtime for their lunch.

This meant that once they got up and, even on Christmas day they get up late, he not only gave them their presents, but a full Christmas lunch for breakfast!

Then they were off to us to open presents. That huge mess of paper on the floor, the reindeer footprints outlined in flour, the piles of presents for the children. The excitement.

Before we went to Sandy's, I had cooked some of the food already, had piles of bowls and plates ready to take across to his house.

While everyone did Christmassy things in his sitting room, once we got to Sandy's, I cooked the veg, did whatever I did with the prepared turkey breast.

Dash wandered in the garden, barked a bit, generally joined in. The children got very excited by their presents. Wendy laid the table that we used about once a year (usually we sit on the couches to eat.)

Sandy would have pointed out again that the Christmas tree was always decorated by the children in whatever way they wanted and they would have looked at the multicoloured chaos they had created out of tinsel and baubles and grumbled that their mum always spoiled their tree at home by being in charge of it.

I poured Wendy and Sandy their Barolo and served the veg. I was so pleased that Sandy said the veg and the food were superb, cooked just as he wanted, that our prawn marie rose and his egg marie rose were as he wanted.

But by the time it was time to go to Wendy's mum, the children were exhausted and fractious!

Not surprising, as they were about to experience their fourth Christmas event of the day!

I went home after dropping off Wendy and the children. Sandy stayed at home. He was in a wonderful mood and said he would have another glass of wine before going to bed.

The children did not behave at Nana's. Despite the huge effort she had gone to with presents and food, the children could not and would not behave.

Wendy ended up home again with me very early, sad because her mum had gone to so much effort and the children had been so difficult.

But the Christmas meal we will remember was at the Queen of the Loch, a couple of days later.

Peter picked up his mum and dad and we arrived all together. I remember we were waiting at the table for quite a time before Sharon arrived but when she did, she came with a buzz of energy and presents and masks for all of us to wear! The children were quickly given a table of their own and sent off to play on the slot machines, well, the catch-a-teddy machines, which was fab because before they had been being quite mutinous but with their own place to sit, slot machines to play with, money, toys, they were in their element.

It was the most lovely time.

There was a hubbub of goodwill and talk and laughter and wondering where we should go to get our food because no one was serving us. Once that was sorted, we ate and talked and laughed.

At some point Sandy said it was the best Christmas he had ever had; the perfect Christmas.

As I write that, I feel some poignancy, but know that when he said it, he was really emphasising this would be his last Christmas, but it also made us very happy to hear it. Very happy that he was able to say that the last Christmas he would have was wonderful, with the people he loved and cared about.

AND WHAT OF THE BEGINNINGS?

These last few years, I have given glimpses into some of the different endings and the beginnings that have accompanied them, but within everything there are beginnings and endings and as far as I can see, rarely can we point to a definite beginning or ending to anything.

I suppose I can't even say I am at the beginning of my relationship with Wendy and the children. When I first met her, she said she had never been in a relationship that lasted longer than seven years and didn't expect to be and so you could say, what of our relationship now that the eighth year is swinging round? It still seems brand new and yet it grows; it also waxes and wanes, changes perspective all the time. We are both terrified that one of us will dump the other which is very reassuring indeed for me; that need to be together.

Our life is full; it is vibrant and exciting but in the most humdrum and lovely of ways. For years we were always up to stuff: cinemas, football, safari parks, wonderful budget holidays, there never seemed to be a pause. Since Covid, that has died down. We still go on holiday but within Scotland, which is maybe better. Last year we stayed in a friend's Airbnb in Easter Ross, in a few weeks we go to another Airbnb in the grounds of a castle in Perthshire. The children do less now, there are fewer chances, but they went to crazy golf and a restaurant on their birthday. Charlotte goes to photography classes, they both have sleepovers. Charlotte has found delight in drawing and writing, James still flourishes with his gaming where he probably meets more people than the rest of us.

For years we went to Fritha and Ffinlo for drunkenness and silliness, every other week. Walking up the long, narrow track in the cold and the dark, half expecting a murderer to leap out at us from the woods; walking up the track in the amber and the pink of the setting sun, walking up the track when the horses are leaning their heads on the gate and the lapwings tumbling in the sky, walking up the track hand in hand, pausing for kisses, walking up the track only holding each other by our pinkies as we are too hot and sweaty.

I have got to know Wendy's friends, who stretch way back into her childhood. I have sat in Jules' garden, sat at McCool's Bar, named after her dog; drinking cocktails, eating my specially made veggie food. I have learned some of her friends' history and witnessed some of the relationships that have disintegrated and some of the relationships that have developed. I have performed in front of them in Helensburgh library when reading my book, *START*, and heard many of the stories of their own beginnings and endings.

And what do we do nowadays? I tend to get up at 7.20, put the coffee and toast on, text Wendy to see what she wants on her toast, call her later to persuade her to get out of bed. I will hear her coming downstairs, hear her delight at seeing Dash at the lookout station he likes to sit at in the mornings and then she will come into the kitchen in her dressing gown for a kiss and a cuddle. Then the sudden motion at 8.00: get dressed, make the lunch, empty the dishwasher while Wendy wakes the children, persuades them to get dressed. The rigamarole of finding out what they want for breakfast. Wendy putting their shoes on while they stare at their iPads, brushing Charlotte's hair, getting them to do their teeth; coats on, bags on, water bottles, Dash on the lead, then a straggle of us down the street, with lots of wittering, often laughter, sometimes squabbles, until we leave them at the corner where Charlotte stops to give us both a big hug and then runs to catch up James who will already be some way up the hill. Before, we would then disappear to trains and work but now we return home. I go upstairs to the bedroom for my tiny desk where I do my Zoom calls (and my bed for when I prefer to work in comfort.) Wendy goes to the sitting room to work in front of the telly.

I still tend to do too much work. I used to be all over Scotland, visiting groups and hospitals, that sort of thing. Now it is more often Zoom calls and some early morning mask-clad, covid-tested visits to hospital wards, and more recently, many, many early morning Zoom calls to professors and academics and the like, around the world, to work out the intricacies of how to make the ideal of international human rights and mental health work in a good way in reality.

Wendy usually has some grand scheme on the go. It may be getting the lop-eared rabbits, doing the Kilt Walk, buying sundials, visiting animal sanctuaries or castles, going on a new diet or anything at all, really. Something is always happening. We could be picking blackberries, walking the Stoneymullen, visiting Juliet for a walk or Peter and Sharon and Clare, David and the children. I might be visiting my mum or doing an online author event. The children might be making cakes or quills out of swan and gull feathers, or they might be playing Pokemon. Charlotte might be absorbed in her book, James might be demanding crisps.

I might be grumbling that the shed is far too full of junk, or grumbling about the state of the car, or complaining about the driveway which I have left full of weeds. We might be planning to go the charity shop in Clydebank where we can leave Dash in the car while we rummage inside.

It is a routine life. For us, every moment is interesting, for many other people it would be like looking at poor holiday snaps, which disguise all the complexity and wonder of living; the things that mean Charlotte loves to spend hours drawing portraits with her mum; James playing on his Xbox and eating supernoodles.

Dash will leap up at us when we have a kiss in the morning. I grumble about tidiness and food and yet rely on Wendy to think of the meals I will cook.

And over the last few years, have I learnt anything? I have, but I have learnt nothing startling. Nothing that means you will say, "Of course, I am so glad to have learnt that from Graham,", but maybe the obviousness of it is a little reassuring.

I have mainly learnt things from Wendy and her dad and her friends, and from relatives. Things like family is important, kindness is important, that there is no need to prove a point for pride's sake. That there is no set way to deal with death, no set formula for grief; there is no textbook for how to express or not express emotion.

I have learnt from my dad and Wendy's dad that sometimes it really 'is what it is'.

The 'let's just get on with it' sort of thing, the acceptance sort of thing.

My life is extraordinarily privileged compared to so many of my friends and the people I work with. If I look around me, I first of all see the awards on the bookshelf, the sculpture Jo George gave me when last I was in hospital, the wooden bedside lamp we got in a charity shop that makes such a soft glow at night, the fragrance diffusers and the ornaments from Crail. The poetry books and the photos of family, the handpainted pictures I got from friends and outside, the pond in the garden, the trampoline our neighbours gave us.

I grumble sometimes about my wages, grumble that I cannot think of anything more responsible than reviewing our legislation and yet I just get my wages that I have lost from the Commission replaced, with no sick leave, holidays, insurance, and the need to do my tax returns every year, but Wendy now works more hours and we can afford odds and ends with ease. We may get almost everything we buy from charity shops, but we do not worry about the food we buy, we feel free to turn the fire on anytime we are cold. I may not buy malt whisky but I am never short of a drink. I may have a very cheap car but I have one. We may have got our dog for free because we are foster carers not owners, but we can afford to pay pet insurance and do not worry about buying him food. We can buy the children presents, take them out on trips, take them to the cinema.

I still worry about what would happen if one of us lost our job and still hope that we can both sell the houses we are renting out so that we can pay off our own mortgage; feel some sort of sense of security. Many of my friends don't have that security. Neither the security of feeling confident about their next meal or the heating bill, nor confident about when next they will speak to someone, when next they will get a hug.

And my work. More and more, I grow weary of some of it. I love it but it seems an impossible task. Sometimes I wonder why we strive, month after month, for change for something better when sometimes we know nothing will make life better. The damage is done, the sadness engrained. I wonder why I do not stamp my feet when you see the same ideas being recycled into the latest fashionable package, just using different words and that optimism people have! That extraordinary belief people can have, that at last they have the answer to mental anguish. Even if there was a definitive cure for mental illness, it would not stop the fact that for many of us despair is still inevitable. Just look at the conflicts, the terrible lives so many people live, the changes to our environment; neither anti-depressants nor comradeship will overcome these issues.

And so many terribly angry people, many of whom are part of a community I was once a part of. I don't understand that anger any more. I know that once, I too felt it. That indignation at injustice, indeed the insistence that our anger was a righteous anger. And that need, both to blame and to keep a tight hold of my own oppression, to explain why I was the way I was. That need to be different and marginalised, that need to be outspoken, individual; to live my own life the way I want.

For many people, my ambition is now something that they would sneer at. I want a job that gives me enough of an income that I can help support my new family, that means I can afford to visit my mum when safe to do so. I do want to see if we can get a better deal for people with a mental illness but I am not going to demonise other people in order to have my say and I am not going to believe there is any one model or answer to such things.

I hate to say it, but I think I am increasingly anti-ambition, anti-changing the world, anti trying to be clever. I fear that people with the latest vision are more likely to cause harm than good. I even worry about individuality and the celebration of difference. I hear that advert 'Dare to be Different'. I have no idea who it is by, and think to myself that that is so much of a con. Wendy helped me question that. Talked about her children and how being different results in exclusion and bullying, whether that is by appearance or behaviour or any of a hundred different things. And it is true, you can see it in the tales from the playground. Those children who do not fit in, who never quite grasped how to play and communicate, they so often are the ones that drift away, get ignored, start that lonely, harsh journey that lacks the dreams that most people growing up have.

I have always been different, it is who I am. I am lucky in that I have been different in a way that people don't seem to find offensive. But when I think about this, I so wish I could have fitted in and belonged. I have never in my life been part of a chattering, excited, joyful crowd of children or adults and I so wish I could have been, that I knew how to do things like that. Part of it was from a basic fear of, I'm not sure what, seeming stupid, getting it wrong and part of it is that I still cannot speak. Not properly, and I wish I knew how to explain this. Put me in an author event, or ask me to give a speech or facilitate a group of people and I can shine and I can charm, but put me in a pub, at a party, put me with my family and my friends and so often, I am not only silent but I have just nothing at all to say. It is not that I have no wish to speak, it is that I am blank and empty of thoughts, empty of anything that might stimulate a conversation and what have the last three years taught me about this?

I think they have taught me that it doesn't matter, though I struggle to actually accept that. For all my silence, for all the crashing boredom I can stimulate, the lack of smiles and all this, Wendy still tells me she loves me and I haven't a clue why. She tells me it is because she fancies me, that despite my claims to be evil, I am kind and gentle and provide some sort of stability in her life. And Wendy's group of girlfriends, they seem to have accepted me, to think of me in a good way and the ex-sisters-in-law, they want our company, and the nephews and nieces, some of them go to special efforts to speak with me.

It makes me very uneasy to say this, but I generally seem to be liked despite my difference. I am not certain enough of that to think I will make new friends in my own right any time soon and to be honest, even as I write this, I want to delete, delete, as it seems so patently absurd. However, maybe after a lifetime of hiding myself away, staring balefully at the happy people and both hating them and wishing to be like them, I find that first of all I no longer hate them and no longer need to aspire to that state. I may one day dare just to be me.

And changing the world, as you see in my mental health posts? Yes, of course, let's do it, but let us remember that just using anger is not an act of morality. So many, many people are full of anger and use it to pursue causes that they will do almost anything to achieve and sacrifice almost anything too. That is not changing the world, that is attacking a world that has damaged you. The individual path towards greatness? Fine. Some people may become famous, may achieve great things despite themselves. My aim, despite my sometimes overbearing individuality, is to learn the art of co-operation and community and belonging.

When I have learnt to give and to treasure and to celebrate, and wonder at the joys and achievements of those around me, then I can change the world, and the world will begin to change around me and whether those favours are returned to me does not matter. I think when I see particularly vile comments on Twitter and instead of getting angry, try to work out why they were made, when I meet people at work, who in the wreckage of their lives strike out at everyone around them and I learn how to give them the equivalent of a welcome hug they would usually shrink from, then I think maybe I am getting somewhere.

But I have so far to go. I managed, a few years ago just before Sandy went into hospital, at the interactive room in Clydebank where I was able to try to dance in front of the children and Wendy and complete strangers, when dancing is the biggest of no-nos for me.

It is these little steps that make a difference. One day, I will be able to swear in front of the family, at least once in a blue moon, just to see the delight on their faces that they have got Graham, the non-swearer to swear.

That is my wisdom. Such a tiny, tiny speck of wisdom. To live that ordinary life and know I am blessed, to see that fame and praise are unnecessary, to know that whatever I achieve at work, in this weird world of rights and justice, it will never be as important or as impressive compared to making Wendy happy, loving the children, walking the dog, sitting on that rock by the Clyde listening to the birds, the wind and the sea. To know there is no need to mark all the beginnings and endings, that is just another form of meaningless achievement. Again, as my dad said, and Sandy said, "It is what it is."

Much of this book has been about the deaths of my dad and Sandy and our reactions to those. When I started writing this book, I was aware there are probably many, very vocal people in the world who write about the theory and reality of dying, grief and bereavement. I have avoided looking at any of these theories or ideas or even ideals, as I said, I am wary of them. I am aware of similar people in my own field of mental health and mental illness and not particularly impressed by the shrill need to convince other people about what to think and do, and I did not want to learn about it in this world of death that every one of us will visit.

The intensity of these years has affected us all profoundly in our tiny family, or perhaps more accurately, our very large melded family. Witnessing death has made dying slightly less frightening, seeing the love people have has thrilled me. Getting to know my dad and Sandy better via their deaths has been such a gift and has helped me to get to know them and myself so much better. I do not necessarily like what I see, but for me, just being able to acknowledge that I can be a pain to be around or work with, is maybe the first positive step in some sort of new story I can only just guess at, at the moment.

It is three p.m. and getting dark. I was awake at three a.m. too, listening to the World Service, hearing people on *Outlook*, finding out the incredible achievements and lives people have had. I had woken to it from a dream that I was a werewolf being hunted down and woke shaking, frightened to move, alert to whoever was waiting in the room for me. I don't expect I will ever escape from my weird terrors or beliefs and to say so, so late in life, that I am getting used to them seems a bit lame, but I think somehow I am.

Wendy still occasionally quotes to the children from a book about how emptying and filling other people's buckets can make them feel, depending on how we treat each other. A simple book we could all learn from. We did a lot of filling Sandy's bucket, as did many other people, and he filled all our buckets. So did my dad. And now they are no longer here, but Dash is lying at my feet, content and fast asleep. Wendy has promised she will try to come on the morning walk with me and Dash, but I imagine she will stay in her bed. The children are at their dad's but we see them in the afternoon, then this bedroom will fill with fluffy toys and I will pull out the sofa bed for the next few days.

It is so trite to say it, but when I watch Wendy talking to strangers in the road, brightening their day, brightening my day, I am struck by all the tiny acts of kindness we can and do give each other and how hard it can be to risk being kind and, although I can't define just what it is, I think the years since I moved to live with Wendy have taught me that

273

the need for kindness and, hard as it is for me to say it, the need for me to be kind to myself is such an important thing.

There are many passages in this story where the hatred I hold for myself shines through. I need to stop relying on my own opinions and start listening to the people around me. Breathe in the joy the world can provide, whether it is through walking with the wind and rain in my face. Snuggling up with Wendy in the evening, cuddling Charlotte at the school gates in the afternoon or smiling when James lets me know he cares for me, despite wishing he had his mum all to himself, all of the time.

My life is mainly good. I will probably yearn for death for all of my life. I will probably be on a section for as long as sections last, but at the same time, I now want to share my wonder at what I have with as many people as I can. That delight that I now belong in Cardross, with this family and a growing number of people that I recognise when I walk to the Co-op for milk in the evening.

As I said to Sandy, "Goodbye, you were a lovely man!" so do I say the same to my dad, who once I hated, and who now I am slowly seeing in a different, brighter, happier light, realising the hatred was more to do with me than him.

Most people are lovely. In fact, if you look hard enough, everyone is lovely and needs treasured. That can be hard sometimes, but everyone can flourish with a little kindness, however trite and sickly that may sound, and however hard it can be to love them when they do all they can to be unloveable. I need to learn that when I am grumbling to myself about imagined slights on one of my windy, chilly winter walks.

Glossary

CPN: A registered nurse who works in the community as part of a team, seeing patients with mental health needs, in various settings.

CTO: Community-based Compulsory Treatment Order: A compulsory treatment order authorises the detention in hospital and/or treatment of a person in the community for a period of six months initially and then for one year at a time.

Depot injection: Long-acting depot injections are used for maintenance therapy, especially when compliance with oral treatment is unreliable.

Detained under the Mental Health Act (sectioned): Being 'sectioned' is the term that is often used when someone is detained under the Mental Health Act. The Mental Health Act is the law which can allow someone to be admitted, detained (or kept) and treated in hospital against their wishes.

Mental Health Tribunal: An independent organisation set up to make decisions on the compulsory care and treatment of people with mental disorders in Scotland.

MHO: A social worker who has special training and experience in working with people who have a mental illness, learning disability or related condition.

Psychiatrist: A physician who specialises in the prevention, diagnosis, and treatment of mental illness.

Psychologist: A mental health professional with highly specialised training in the diagnosis and psychological treatment of mental, behavioural and emotional illness.

Acknowledgements

This book was hardly a book before my editor, Clare Cain, got her hands on it. Her ability to get me to delete and delete has made this into something I am very proud of. Thank you so much, Clare, and thanks also to all those people who looked at and tried to comment on various drafts – I hope I have included everyone! Ailsa Crum, Aine Kennedy, Vicki Souter, Tom Brown, Cynthia Rogerson, Joanna Higgs, Carolyn Papakyriakou, Mary Mowat, Maggie Wallis and John and Cath King.

'I took three months off sick because of my mental ill-health and had the most fun in ages' was first published on Mental Health Today – www.mentalhealthtoday.co.uk.

'Short break at Knockderry Castle' was originally published in PENning magazine, 2020.

'Reality Check' was originally written for the Scottish Mental Health Arts Festival.

'When life was kinder: reflections of a disillusioned mental health activist' was first published on Mental Health Today – www.mentalhealthtoday.co.uk.

'Storytelling as an agent of change' was first published on Psychreg – www.psychreg.org.

Some thoughts on *Blackbird Singing*

Graham Morgan nails it again – grief, confusion, surprise, romantic love and delight, all wrapped up in poetic observations. I could read his work all day. His best book yet.

--Cynthia Rogerson, author of *I Love You, Goodbye, Wah!: Things I Never Told My Mother* and others.

Graham's wonderful story of managing love, death, work and mind, provides 'no answers and no truths,' but instead provides the reader with a disarming and tender reflection on a life impacted by serious mental illness – simply locating sublime moments of beauty, meaning and joy in the events of his everyday life.

--Linda Gask, writer and psychiatrist.

Graham warmly invites us to accompany him through the daily joys and struggles of family life, his dreams and nightmares. As he reflects on the impact of his mental ill-health, he draws us close. We care for those he cares for so deeply; his partner, the children, friends and family and Dash, the dog. As a reader you feel alongside him, walking in the rain, sailing choppy seas, snuggled up before a fire, sharing a dram. Fathers figure large; his own, his partner's and himself as a father. Sometimes brutally honest, always exploring the wonder of his environment and the people around him, Graham lays before us the excruciating challenges of being human; of love, of death, of forgiveness and understanding. Beautifully and lovingly written.

--Alison Bavidge, National Director, Scottish Association of Social Work.

Blackbird Singing is a personal story of family and loss. Graham shares his thoughts, especially during the period of Covid lockdown, and gives us vivid images of those he loves and has loved. We see glimpses of the often debilitating impact of his intense self-reflection and insight into his illness. His stories are set against a backdrop of nature which offers a constant and reassuring canvas for the tears, laughter and cuddles.

Despite some intense lows and recent losses, as Graham says, "I am still here and I still smile and I still love, despite my lack of practice at it. Despite my fear that I will never get it right."

--John Scott QC Solicitor Advocate, Chair, Scottish Mental Health Law Review.